CARCINOID CANCER, ZEBRAS AND STARDUST

My sister's cancer battle

CARCINOID CANCER, ZEBRAS AND STARDUST

My sister's cancer battle

Mary Girsch-Bock

Unlimited Publishing LLC
Bloomington, Indiana

ISBN
Paperback:1-58832-162-2
Hard Cover:1-158832-163-0
Library of Congress Control Number 2006934495

Unlimited Publishing LLC
Bloomington, Indiana

http://www.unlimitedpublishing.com
author web site: www.stardustcreations.net

Acknowledgments

This book would not exist without the extraordinary assistance provided by Dr. Eugene Woltering M.D. and Dr. Lowell Anthony M.D. of Louisiana State University Health Sciences Center in Kenner, Louisiana. Both were willing to take the time to educate a total stranger about Carcinoid Cancer. A special thanks also goes to Dr. Woltering for being kind enough to edit the completed manuscript for medical accuracy. You have my untold admiration and gratitude.

I'd also like to thank Jack Magestro at Unlimited Publishing, whose expertise has made this experience enjoyable.

To Kathy Wright and Carol-Anne Wilson, who, from the beginning, have been so supportive of my efforts to write about my sister's carcinoid journey. Thank you.

To Tom and Vicki Bee, who six years ago were my employers, but are now family. Thank you for your support and for being an inspiration to me.

To the Carcinoid Cancer Foundation and The Caring For Carcinoid Foundation for working tirelessly to educate patients and the medical community about this rare disease.

I'd also like to thank The Carcinoid Cancer Foundation for granting me permission to draw from their vast collection of medical data during the writing of this book.

To Jesse Tyminski, the rock that Marge frequently leaned on. You are and always will be family.

A heartfelt thanks to my friend Donna Blizniak for being there when I needed you, and to my lifelong friend Fran Parker, whose friendship has been and remains one of the most important things in my life.

To my son Jared, who is the most intelligent, compassionate, sensitive, and funny eight year old I have ever met, and to my husband Shannon, whose seemingly endless supply of love and patience has nurtured me through some of the best and worst days of my life, and whose continuous support throughout the writing of this book and after, means more than I can ever say. I love you both forever.

Finally, a thank you to all those carcinoid patients who continue to battle this disease with a level of strength, dignity, and determination that is astounding. You were an inspiration to my sister Marge, and continue to be an inspiration to me as well. May you all receive the care you deserve.

Note

The Zebra is the unofficial mascot of the carcinoid community. Taken from the old medical school analogy "If you hear hoof beats, think horses," carcinoid patients, their family and friends want you to know that sometimes it's not a horse you hear. Sometimes it's a zebra.

Carcinoid IS cancer. This is something that I believe is important for everyone to know and understand, from those in the medical community, to the average citizen. If more people become aware of this disease, the odds that future carcinoid patients receive the correct treatment improve dramatically. Knowledge is power, as most carcinoid patients know. Sometimes it can even save a life. Please take the time to learn about this disease.

Mary Girsch-Bock – April 2006

To my big sister
Marge
1956 - 2004

I Miss You

TABLE OF CONTENTS

INTRODUCTION

Stardust Memories

It's early May, and I'm sitting here on the seventh floor balcony of the Stardust Hotel. I'm here with my sister Marge, whose favorite place in the world is Las Vegas, and the Stardust in particular. It's about an hour before sunrise, and I'm wide-awake.

Inside our room, Marge is sleeping, having lasted admirably until nearly 4:00 AM. I say 'admirably' because she is dying of something called carcinoid cancer; a disease that has slowly robbed her of her vitality and strength, and will eventually end her life.

But throughout her illness, she has always managed to get to Las Vegas. In this town of make believe, we can pretend that everything is the same as it used to be, if only for a short time.

And pretend we do.

Our evening is spent at a Las Vegas show, a limousine ride to Marge's favorite Italian restaurant, and then gambling until 3:00 AM.

I take a deep breath, enjoying the cool air, and the smell of jasmine wafting up from the lush gardens below. The scent is calming after a night spent in smoky casinos.

May has always been our favorite month in Las Vegas. Late spring blossoms are at their peak; their last hurrah before the brutal summer heat arrives. Perhaps, like Marge, they are aware that their time is running out. Maybe that's why they are so musky and fragrant tonight. In the pre-dawn hours, jasmine, gardenia, rose, and honeysuckle all blend together to form a fragrance that is uniquely Las Vegas. The scent surrounds me, bringing me peace.

Marge's birthday is in May; the only month you can truly enjoy the natural beauty of the desert. May is a month of warm days and cool nights, where the grass is still a virgin green, pale and delicate. The palm trees are lush and exotic, with full foliage that poufs delicately like the crown of a surprised cockatoo. Soon the pale green grass will darken until, by August, it will be parched and withered, with rough, straw-like patches scattered throughout. Palm trees will droop in the mid-afternoon heat. They will only perk up when the sun has set.

I know that when August nears, the desert scent that now permeates my senses will be gone. What else will be gone?

I breathe deeply, trying to store the scent, and this trip in my memory.

As dawn breaks over the mountains to the east, another day begins. The birds are louder now, more insistent. As the sun rises higher over the Las Vegas valley, their chirping will lessen. Sunrise in Las Vegas has a spiritual overtone. If there were a perfect time to pray, it would be right now.

So I pray. I pray that my sister will beat the odds and that we will be here next year, watching the sunrise together. In early morning Las Vegas, I pray for a miracle. Indigo skies are gradually lightening, as the faint outline of the mountains surrounding Las Vegas gradually take shape, their purplish blue hue forming a perimeter around the valley.

This is Las Vegas at its most vulnerable; when the bold, brassy, beckoning lights cannot entice the unsuspecting visitor quite so effectively. Against the ever-lightening sky, the casinos look harmlessly festive and innocuous, their bright neon reduced to a faint twinkle.

Yes, this is our favorite time in Las Vegas, when the raucous meets the relaxed, each having its own virtues. If I closed my eyes, I could imagine myself somewhere in the tropics. But at this particular moment, I can honestly say that there is no other place that I would rather be than where I am right now.

I turn back to look at Marge sleeping peacefully. As I look at the sun rising over Sunrise Mountain, I am happy that we can greet another day together. How many more we will share, I don't know. Today, we won't think about the future. We'll just enjoy our favorite city one more day.

Five months later, my sister, Margaret 'Marge' Durlak passed away from a pancreatic carcinoid tumor. Marge fought this tumor every day of her life since she was diagnosed in 1995. She was just beginning to have confidence in herself professionally and still had many goals left to accomplish at the time of her death. One thing is for certain; Marge did not want to die.

What she did want was information. Lots of information. What is a carcinoid tumor? How is a diagnosis of carcinoid different from a traditional cancer diagnosis? What could she do to stop the debilitating diarrhea that she suffered from on a daily basis? What could she do to stop the pain?

These are just a few of the questions she had. Unfortunately, most of these questions remained unanswered at the time of her death. Even the doctors treating her did not have any answers.

The sad fact is that few physicians even see a carcinoid patient during their entire professional career. Those that do often operate under the mistaken notion that once diagnosed, the patient need only be monitored for tumor growth. The "if it ain't broken, don't fix it" premise is frequently practiced by physicians, many who are reluctant to subject patients with 'manageable symptoms' to the side effects that more aggressive treatment may invoke.

While this 'wait and see' approach can be the correct course of treatment in many patients, others with a more aggressive tumor will suffer the consequences of this treatment delay later on down the road.

Many of my sister's friends and colleagues had no idea just how sick she was. Most viewed carcinoid as many would an ulcer; painful, debilitating, but certainly not life threatening.

The idea for this book came to light the night of Marge's memorial service. Many of her friends arrived in shock, unable to comprehend her death. "What was the name of that disease again?" "What is carcinoid?" And "wasn't there anything that could be done?" Time after time, I was asked these questions, many of which I was unable to answer. Towards the end of the service, I realized two things; that most people have absolutely no idea what carcinoid is, and that there are no quick, easy answers to these questions.

Carcinoid tumors, part of the neuroendocrine tumor family, damage the body by flooding it with excess hormones that are produced by the tumor. These are the same hormones that a healthy endocrine system produces. But the problem is when they are produced in large amounts, they become lethal to the body. Thus patients often suffer more from the symptoms of these tumors, rather than from the spread of tumors as is usually the case in more traditional cancers.

There are a select group of specialists scattered throughout the country who have devoted their lives to researching and treating this disease. The words of many of those specialists can be found throughout this book.

What I want to accomplish with this book is twofold. I wish to share the struggles of my sister Marge, who was and remains the inspiration behind this book. And I want to educate people about this rare and often deadly disease.

My sister so wanted to share her story with others. After struggling with her death, I decided I would do my best to make her desire a reality.

One of the physicians I spoke with shared a quote with me that I often turn to when things get rough: "Out of darkness, God created light. Out of your darkness, you must create a future."

Out of my darkness, this book was created. And if just one person is helped by it, I will have created a future, theirs and mine.

CHAPTER ONE
My Big Sister

Margaret Ann Durlak was born May 8th, 1956. I followed some 16 months later. Because only 16 months separated us, we were very close, even as young children.

We grew up in an apartment about four miles west of Wrigley Field in Chicago. My mother was very protective of us, thus our outside playtime was negligible. We contented ourselves with playing indoor games, or just creating our own.

Neither Marge nor I ever went anywhere without the other. My mother even dressed us alike, so we were frequently asked if we were twins. Mom died when Marge was twelve, and I was ten. Because of her death, we drew even closer together. Forced to grow up quickly, we took over the job of cleaning the house and shopping for groceries while my dad worked.

While we had always fought, as most siblings do, our arguments escalated as we reached our teens. We both were struggling with our own identity, and slowly becoming the people we were meant to be.

Our three-person household was frequently wrought with arguments, mostly between my sister and my dad. They both loved to yell, and their arguments frequently became shouting matches. Neither one held a grudge; usually within ten minutes of an argument, they were talking sweetly to one another.

All this shouting wore me out. When I reached 21, I moved into my own apartment. Marge chose to stay with my dad. During that time, they formed a bond that remained unbroken, even after my father's death in 1996. I believe that bond still exists today, and I'm happy that they are together once again. During the early part of her life, Marge was angry and very defensive. It was very difficult to get close to her; even with the closeness that we shared, she frequently pushed me away. After being diagnosed with carcinoid, her priorities shifted. During the last five years of her life, I saw a dramatic change in her. Always impatient, she learned the art of patience. Often judgmental of others, she learned to be more open, and more forgiving of both her own and other people's shortcomings. And the anger that she carried with her nearly her entire life seemed to dissipate.

Because my dad was estranged from much of his family, we were isolated from many of our aunts, uncles, and cousins. When my half-brother Gary committed suicide, we were only told after his funeral. We had not spoken to my other half-brother Jim in years, and my sister carried tremendous bitterness toward him. But a chance meeting between Marge and Jim at a veterinarian's office brought the two of them together, and five months before she died, we had lunch together, closing all past wounds, and finally reconciling as a family.

There are several reasons why I believe Marge did not seek out more expert help in dealing with carcinoid. I think on one level, she simply did not accept the fact that carcinoid could kill her. I also believe that she had absolute trust in her doctors, and honestly believed that they were doing their best for her. When it became obvious that her health was deteriorating, she made the choice to stick with the doctor who had been treating her, rather than seek out a specialist.

I spoke to one of her home-health nurses several weeks before she died. It was the nurse who told me that Marge was dying. I refused to believe it. But on a certain level I knew it was true. A week later, Jesse called me from the hospital. He had just spoken with Marge's doctor, who had given her two weeks to live.

We immediately made plans to head to Chicago, leaving the following day. We were fifteen minutes from the hospital when Jesse called us to say that Marge had died. She had lasted only three days.

When we arrived at the hospital, I sat in the room, alone, and talked to Marge. I stroked her hair and her face, telling her how sorry I was that I didn't get a chance to say good-bye to her. I was so angry; at her doctors, at the hospital, and at Marge, for dying before we got there.

I have tried somewhat successfully to let some of that anger go. I do believe that her doctors were doing everything that they could. It just wasn't enough.

Marge died September 29th, 2004: the same day, and nearly the same time as my father. Because they were so close in life, I believe my dad was there that day, holding out a hand to her, wanting to end her pain and suffering. Those of us left behind could do nothing other than grieve, and yet be grateful that she was no longer suffering.

Mary Girsch-Bock

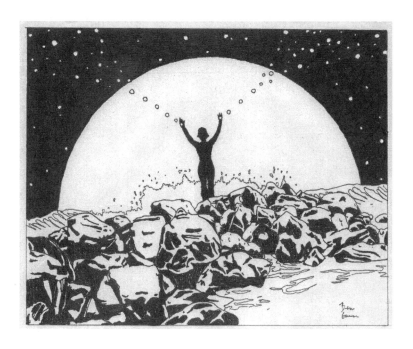

CHAPTER TWO
Carcinoid Confusion

"It all began one fall night in 1985. That night, after going to bed, I experienced a pain in my stomach unlike any other. I got up and took an antacid, but it didn't work. By morning the pain had gone."

—From Marge's Diary

My sister's story, in her words, can be found at the back of this book. Please read it to get a better understanding of what Marge went through on a daily basis. As Marge's sister, I know there is much that she left out. These are small details that only family and close friends would know. Things like how we would go out for dinner, and before we left the restaurant, Marge would be in the restroom, vomiting or having profuse diarrhea. Or the fact that shortly after dinner, we could expect to see her doubled over in pain as she fought to digest her food. None of those things ever stopped her from living her life exactly how she wanted to. Most of the time, she had more energy than many of her friends. From the very beginning, until the very end, whether on vacation, at a party, or during the excitement of the holidays, Marge unequivocally enjoyed her life, perhaps because she was aware of how fragile it was.

Although Marge and I spoke on the telephone every day, sometimes twice, we never really discussed her 'terminal' illness. While our conversations certainly centered on how she was feeling, or my nagging her to seek a more expert medical opinion, Marge was never interested in talking about her mortality. I'm not sure if she just refused to voice it simply because she would then be admitting it, or she was more comfortable keeping it to herself. Whatever the reason, Marge refused to discuss the possibility of dying, and maintained that position until she took her final breath.

Shortly after her tumor was discovered, my dad remarked that Marge was too stubborn to die. I do believe that statement was at least partially true. Marge lived with her tumor for nearly twenty years without any interventional treatment at all save Sandostatin®, which is octreotide acetate, an injectable medication that slows or stops severe diarrhea. She would have died much sooner without this medication.

I cannot tell you with any certainty that Marge would have lived longer had she sought the care of a physician who was experienced in treating carcinoid and neuroendocrine tumors. I suspect that may be true, but it could simply be one of my regrets that I did not fight harder to get her to a more experienced physician. While the decision to seek a new physician (or not) was ultimately Marge's responsibility, I am selfish enough to wish she were still alive today.

Interestingly enough, my sister was able to pinpoint almost to the day, when the symptoms of her pancreatic carcinoid tumor began. In fact, the majority of those eventually diagnosed with a carcinoid tumor have already had the disease for many years prior to a definitive diagnosis. But just what is carcinoid cancer?

Carcinoid tumors belong to a larger group of tumors called neuroendocrine tumors. They develop from enterochromaffin cells, which are found in the lining of the stomach, small, and large intestines, as well as the appendix, rectum, pancreas, lungs, and the liver. Entero means relating to the stomach and chromaffin refers to a silver stain reaction similar to the chromaffin cells that are found in the adrenal glands. The enterochromaffin cells are known to produce 90 percent of the body's supply of serotonin, as well as histamine, dopamine, and tachykinins. Because carcinoid tumors form directly from enterochromaffin cells, they maintain their ability to produce these substances, subsequently flooding the body with massive quantities of hormones that can prove lethal. Normally, this flood of chemicals does not occur unless the primary tumor has metastasized to the liver. For instance, if your primary tumor is located in the small intestine, than any hormones produced by this tumor will flow through the portal vein, which is a large vein that carries blood from the stomach and intestines to the liver. The liver then destroys the hormones before releasing the blood back into general circulation. However, if your primary tumor has metastasized to the liver, the hormones are no longer destroyed by the liver, but instead are released directly into the bloodstream. It's also important to note that if the primary tumor is located in the lungs or ovaries, metastases is not necessary for hormones to be released throughout the body.

Carcinoid tumors are frequently classified as 'functioning,' or 'non-functioning.' It is the functioning tumors that secrete excessive hormones that flood the body and can wreak havoc with everyday life. The type of hormones that a tumor secretes depends on the type of tumor a person has been diagnosed with. Although carcinoid tumors are the most common neuroendocrine tumors, there are others similar to carcinoid that can produce many of the same symptoms. These include Insulinomas, which secrete insulin, Gastrinomas, which secrete excess gastrin, VIPomas, which secrete VIP, and Glucagonomas, which secrete glucagon. Depending on the location of the primary tumor, a carcinoid tumor can secrete any or all of these hormones, along with serotonin, histamine, and chromogranin-A (CgA). Only by performing specialized blood, urine and stain testing can a proper diagnosis be made, and the correct treatment initiated.

Carcinoid is not a new disease. In 1888, pathologist Otto Lubarsch was the first to describe the unique cells found in carcinoid tumors. In 1890, W. B. Ransom went on to define and describe carcinoid syndrome. Finally, in 1907, a German pathologist named Siegfried Oberndorfer introduced the term carcinoid (Karzinoide) in order to distinguish between the more aggressive carcinomas and benign adenomas. Though both tumors looked somewhat alike, their behavior was quite different. And to make an accurate diagnosis even more difficult, these unusual tumors shared characteristics of both carcinomas and adenomas. The resulting name 'carcinoid' means somewhere between malignant and benign.

This is an ideal description of carcinoid, which has often been described in the medical community as 'cancer in slow motion.' Unfortunately many in the medical community have come to categorize these complex tumors as benign, a myth that has been carried forward into twenty first century medicine, frequently to the detriment of those who are unfortunate enough to be diagnosed with one.

Although study after study has shown that indeed carcinoid is not as benign as once thought, the 'wait and see' approach is still frequently employed by even the most experienced physicians, at some of the best hospitals in the United States.   Such was the case with my sister.   She suffered increasingly painful symptoms for nearly ten years before receiving a proper diagnosis. Even after surgery, and analysis by two pathologists, physicians were still unsure about the type of tumor she had. Both normal and abnormal cells were found in the tumor, but without performing the staining procedure mentioned earlier, pathologists were unable to determine what type of tumor she had. It took another year before she was given a definitive diagnosis, and provided any treatment. As 'benign' as many physicians think carcinoid is, it is important to remember that people die from this disease. Of those who do, you can be sure that the majority of them were simply diagnosed too late. It's common knowledge that an early diagnosis and prompt treatment can make all the difference in the world to a cancer patient. That same principle holds true for carcinoid patients as well.

In hindsight, I realize that the pain my sister had that night was just the start of many pain-filled days and nights that went unexplained for years. It's fair to note that those same pains could just as easily been caused by something as simple as indigestion. But when unexplained pain continues for months and years, it is time to look beyond the 'quick fix' and start considering the possibility that a more serious and perhaps rare disease may be the cause of continuous, unrelenting pain.

That first night of pain was only the beginning. Marge would go on to experience numerous 'episodes' as she called them. These episodes would span a decade.

Throughout the years, numerous doctors had the opportunity to locate the cause of Marge's continuous pain, and begin treatment, sooner rather than later. Instead, doctor after doctor pronounced her as 'too fat,' suggested that she lose some weight, told her to stop eating fried foods, and try to cut down on sweets. After these in-depth diagnoses, she was simply sent on her way. There was no concerted effort made to locate the source of her pain. Subsequent visits with the same physicians always elicited the same recommendations. Not one doctor suggested that she go for further testing, or any testing for that matter. Not knowing the medical particulars of her case, other than what she told me, I can only speculate that prompt treatment may have prolonged her life. I'll never know that for sure, but I do know that I would be more accepting of her death at the age of forty-eight if I thought that all possible treatment possibilities had been exhausted.

As Dr. Richard R.P. Warner M.D., Clinical Professor of Medicine at Mount Sinai Hospital in New York City, and Medical Director of the Carcinoid Cancer Foundation said during his talk at the California Carcinoid Fighters conference in October of 2003, "This concept of (carcinoid) being so 'benign' and therefore not worthy of treatment has to be disqualified."

Mary Girsch-Bock

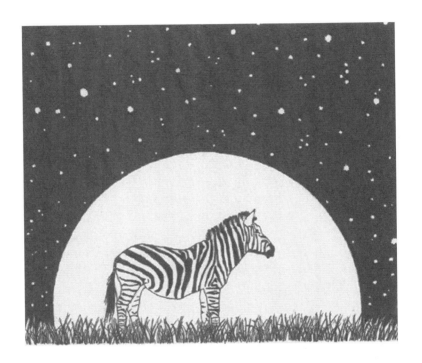

CHAPTER THREE
It's All In Your Head

"I sought the advice of still another doctor, who basically offered me the same advice as all the others. I also received a prescription for Prilosec. I requested an ultrasound of my gallbladder and the doctor finally agreed, but the ultrasound displayed nothing. So I was told to raise the head of my bed, sleep on my right side, and lose more weight. I didn't think being fat could cause this much pain. It was at that moment that I resigned myself to the fact that I was just going to have to live with this pain. I was also beginning to think I was crazy."

—From Marge's Diary

According to Dr. Lowell Anthony MD, Director of Gastrointestinal and Neuroendocrine Oncology, and Associate Professor of Medicine at Louisiana State University Health Sciences Center in New Orleans, LA, many patients admit that their family physician had previously declared their multitude of symptoms 'psychological.' Women, particularly, have this problem, as the symptoms of menopause such as flushing can frequently be similar to the symptoms of a carcinoid tumor producing too many hormones. However, there is one difference between the flushing experienced by a woman in menopause, and a woman with carcinoid. If the flushing is 'wet' (accompanied by heavy perspiration), it usually means the cause of the flushing does not originate from the neuroendocrine system. If the flush is 'dry' (no perspiration), it most likely originates from the neuroendocrine system.

Marge began noticing a pattern in her symptom flare-ups. They all occurred around her menstrual cycle. When mentioning this to her doctor, it was dismissed as unrelated. But Dr. Anthony disagrees. "The increased hormone production that occurs around a women's menstrual cycle can definitely cause an increase in the symptoms of carcinoid."

Dr. Anthony goes on to state that some women have resorted to having a hysterectomy because their symptoms were so debilitating.

This multitude of inexplicable symptoms is usually what drives patients to eventually seek medical attention. These symptoms can include unexplained pain, flushing, wheezing and, most prominently, diarrhea. Many patients also suffer from unexplained fatigue, and weight loss. A physician even remotely acquainted with carcinoid may begin to question these symptoms and order the appropriate tests (which will be discussed later) in order to rule out carcinoid. But for physicians who have never treated a patient with a carcinoid tumor, this option will not be presented. Instead, standard diagnostic testing will most likely be done, which may or may not pinpoint a carcinoid tumor. When these diagnostic tests continue to come back with normal levels, as they often do, a diagnosis of depression becomes almost understandable. As I mentioned earlier, Marge was repeatedly advised to lose weight. For nearly ten years, she was given this advice from a variety of doctors who were unable to see past the picture she presented: an overweight woman who looked healthy. No further testing was deemed necessary.

As time went on, it gradually became easier for Marge to believe that the problem was psychological. When you are told over and over again that there is nothing wrong with you, yet you continue to experience the same pain, it becomes easier to believe that the problem may be 'all in your head.' It was at that time that Marge decided she needed to learn to live with the pain.

I have difficulty remembering a time when Marge was not in pain. At first it was sporadic; an upset stomach here, some pain there. Certainly nothing to be concerned about. But over time the frequency and the intensity increased. What used to be a 'once a month' pain, became a weekly pain, then a daily pain. For the last five years of her life, Marge was in daily pain, with the pain beginning in her upper abdomen and shooting like a knife into her back. Always present, the pain intensified after meals. Marge usually managed to hide it well, but those close to her knew better. Strangely enough, the only thing that would make her pain less intense was hanging her upper body down toward the floor. Her "hanging" as she called it, became a regular occurrence after each meal. It looked painful to me, but it was the only thing that would reduce the pain of digesting her meals.

Unexplained pain is an obvious sign that something is wrong. When coupled with the seemingly endless search for a doctor who will pay attention to your symptoms, frustration and depression can certainly come into play. Unfortunately, frustration and depression are what doctors first noticed when they saw Marge. As a result, they never looked beyond that to find the source of her pain.

It's also important to remember that a Carcinoid tumor does not make anyone's top ten list of possible diagnosis. Or even the top twenty. In fact, Dr. Warner suggests that the reason why many carcinoid sufferers go undiagnosed for so long is because many physicians simply do not even 'think' of carcinoid when searching for answers. Because of the relative rarity of carcinoid and neuroendocrine tumors (approximately 8,000 are diagnosed each year) this holds true even if many of the telltale signs and symptoms of carcinoid present themselves (constant diarrhea, flushing, pain). It simply does not occur to physicians to test for it. Statistics have shown that the majority of carcinoid tumors are discovered during surgery for unspecified abdominal pain or after patients develop a bowel obstruction from a progressing tumor.

If a carcinoid tumor is suspected, a blood test called a Chromogranin-A level (CgA) screening can be done. Chromogranin A is a protein that is secreted into the circulatory system by neuroendocrine tumors, including carcinoid tumors. CgA levels will usually be elevated if a carcinoid tumor is present.

Another test that can be done is the 5-HIAA-urine test. But while an elevated 5-HIAA level can often help in confirming a carcinoid diagnosis, not all carcinoid patients will have elevated 5-HIAA levels.

But the real problem continues to be awareness. If the physician does not even consider carcinoid as a possible diagnosis, they will not be running either of these tests.

CHAPTER FOUR
It's NOT All In Your Head

"It was now 1992. The pain was happening more frequently and with greater intensity. I was now vomiting and having more frequent bowel movements on a regular basis. My attacks, when they happened, were lasting twenty four to forty eight hours. During an attack I was unable to eat or drink anything."

—From Marge's Diary

It was clear that Marge's symptoms were not disappearing. H2 blockers such as Zantac and Pepcid were not reducing or eliminating her pain. It was also clear that her symptoms were too severe to ignore. After demanding further testing, Marge was sent for an Upper GI Series, an Ultrasound of the Gallbladder, and an Endoscope. The tests revealed nothing out of the ordinary. A doctor familiar with carcinoid tumors, aware of the symptoms that Marge presented, might have suggested testing 5-HIAA or CgA levels at this time.

I remember being with Marge during many of her severe attacks. It was impossible for her to eat anything. Even a sip of water caused her to gag. She spent days doubled over in pain, swallowing Advil like candy. Her frustration and mine continued to grow. How could anyone be in such unmitigating pain and yet be told time and again that there was 'nothing wrong?'

Either the doctors were wrong or Marge was.

But I had seen firsthand the effect these attacks had on her. I saw the pain etched in her face, her eyes dull and lifeless.

Marge was not wrong.

So we continued on our quest for answers.

In early 1994, Marge approached yet another doctor. After pouring out ten years of pain and frustration, this doctor did not suggest she lose weight, eat less fried foods, or sleep with her head elevated. She sent her for an MRI.

The MRI revealed a mass near her pancreas. A subsequent biopsy revealed both normal and abnormal cells. It is not unusual in carcinoid to find both types of cells present. Remember, carcinoid is cancer; but cancer in slow motion. The cells do not divide at the same rate as those found in routine carcinomas.

But the presence of both types of cells puzzled my sister's doctor, who eventually blamed the findings on lab errors. This information clearly signaled the need for further testing to rule out carcinoid. Again, no carcinoid testing was done.

Marge was relieved that something had been found; yet devastated about the presence of a tumor on her pancreas. Her physician referred her to a surgeon for an evaluation. Not comfortable with the first surgeon, Marge sought out a second opinion. On a recommendation from a hospital colleague, she made an appointment with a surgeon at a major teaching hospital in Chicago. The surgeon, an affable man with a confident air jokingly told her during her initial exam "if this tumor were malignant, you would have been dead years ago."

I suppose this should have been reassuring, and at the time it was. But in retrospect, I find it arrogant, and narrow-minded, and exactly the attitude that so many carcinoid patients frequently find in their quest for answers.

Thankfully, the vast majority of physicians treat their patients with kindness and respect. These are the same physicians that call carcinoid specialists for a consultation, and are open to educating themselves about carcinoid and neuroendocrine tumors including the proper testing, and treatment options that are available.

But to many in the medical field, the common refrain remains; if they're slow growing, what's the hurry?

The hurry is that if a patient is diagnosed early, and the tumor removed, the chance of future metastases goes way down. If a tumor is removed early enough, patients can frequently be considered cured. However, when the tumors are left remaining in the body, even a 'slow-growing' tumor can eventually metastasize to the liver, or other sites throughout the body, including the lungs, bone, or even the brain. Tumors left in the body can also entwine around major arteries, press on major organs, or cause intestinal obstructions.

In May of 1994, Marge had surgery at a major teaching hospital in Chicago. However, like everything else, the surgery did not go according to plan. Once the surgeon made the incision, a piece of the tumor was cut away and sent to pathology for a diagnosis. But as before, the lab was unable to accurately diagnose the tumor type.

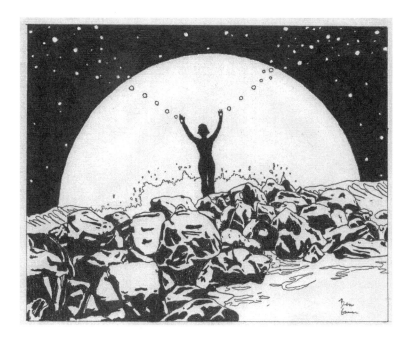

CHAPTER FIVE
The Surgery That Never Was

"As I said my goodbyes, I knew in my gut that this tumor would still be with me after surgery."

—*From Marge's Diary*

Remember the last time you caught the flu? The day before you knew you were getting sick, yet you had no true symptoms, no fever, no aches or pains. You just knew you were getting sick. We all know our own bodies better than anyone else, even the most competent physician. Marge knew prior to surgery that the tumor would not be removed. I will never be able to tell you how she knew this, but she did.

Once again, the lab was not able to accurately confirm the type of tumor. Unable to proceed without a definitive diagnosis, the surgeon declined to remove the tumor, and abruptly ended the surgery, thus proving Marge correct.

At the time of Marge's surgery, I was living nearly two thousand miles away in Nevada. I sat by the phone all day, impatiently waiting for word from my Dad or Marge's boyfriend Jesse about how the surgery had gone. As the minutes turned to hours, I tried to remain calm, but I finally picked up the phone.

Still nothing.

Late in the afternoon, Jesse finally called. He was crying. My hand clenched the phone as my heart thumped loudly in my chest.

"What's wrong?" I yelled in his ear, but he didn't respond.

"What's wrong?" I asked again, trying to remain calm, but failing miserably.

"The doctor said there was nothing they could do."

What did that mean? Suddenly I remembered back to when I was ten and my mother was diagnosed with cancer.

My father had used those exact words; 'there's nothing they could do.'

"They didn't take it out?" I asked. I found that odd, since I had been with Marge during her exam with the surgeon, and he had been confident that they could remove the tumor without a problem.

"He said they couldn't," Jesse told me.

Silence.

I tried to comprehend Jesse's words. I tried to process the information in my mind, but I refused to face the reality that those words conjured up. 'There was nothing they could do?' This was from the cocky surgeon who two weeks earlier predicted a smooth, uncomplicated procedure?

But Jesse wasn't finished.

"He said that the tumor was also in her liver."

It was in the liver? To my knowledge, benign tumors didn't spread to the liver.

"Does Marge know?" I asked.

"No," said Jesse. "No one's told her."

CHAPTER SIX
Wait…and Wait…and See

"When I finally woke up it was 5:30 in the afternoon. They were just about ready to take me to my room. I saw both my dad and Jesse in the hall as they were wheeling me through. They both looked pretty bad. When I finally got into bed, I asked Jesse if I was dying. He said no. So I told both Jesse and my dad to get that look off of their faces."
                                                    —From Marge's Diary

The next day, the surgeon came in to visit my sister during rounds. He told her that he did not remove the tumor. Unfortunately, he was unable to answer most of Marge's questions. He just didn't know. He went on to tell her that he had made an appointment for her with an oncologist that specialized in pancreatic tumors. It was at that point that Marge simply stopped listening. She was trying to process two things: the fact that she had a pancreatic tumor, and that she would be seeing an oncologist. No other words were spoken during that visit, but from the tone, and the foreboding look on his face, Marge's main impression was that the prognosis was grim.

Marge spent the next week thinking nothing but the worst. The surgeon, having delivered his devastating news to Marge, subsequently washed his hands of her and her tumor.

Two weeks later, Marge met with the oncologist. After the meeting, she said she felt better. The oncologist explained to her that they would simply monitor the tumor, and if it showed any signs of growth, she would have to undergo chemotherapy. He scheduled her next CT scan in two months. When she went for her first post-operative CT scan, there was no change, so they scheduled her for another scan in three months.

Eventually, Marge's care was turned over to another oncologist. She continued to have scans done every three months. No one ever explained to Marge what type of tumor she had, just that it was a pancreatic tumor. Treatment options were never discussed, and no medication was ever suggested or prescribed.

Marge had returned home from the hospital much the same as she had been before the surgery. Her tumor, her nausea, her vomiting, and her pain were still there, as was a new addition, the six-inch scar across her abdomen.

Nothing had changed.

But unbeknownst to Marge, something had changed.

CHAPTER SEVEN
New Symptoms

"Shortly after my surgery, I noticed that I began having strange diarrhea. But because the CT scans showed no difference in my tumor size, the doctor didn't think it was related. I didn't mention it again

At the end of the year, my oncologist informed me that he was moving to Springfield, Illinois. I had grown comfortable with him and was concerned about where my treatment would go. Little did I know that on my next visit I would meet the doctor who would finally diagnose and treat my disease."

—From Marge's Diary

Within a few weeks of visiting her new oncologist, Marge found her diarrhea worsening. The diarrhea was now accompanied by nausea and weakness. Even so, Marge forced herself to go to work every morning. She had just spent six weeks off recovering from surgery, and she didn't want to spend any additional time away from work. It wasn't easy. She found herself having a difficult time staying awake during the day, and her muscles had taken on a strange ache. Each day, she found herself growing weaker and weaker. By the end of the day, she could barely climb the stairs at home. Soon, even walking became nearly impossible. Her doctor prescribed some medication for the nausea, but it didn't really work. Her diarrhea continued, as she grew even weaker.

This continued on for over a month. In September of 1995, she lost 45 pounds. Her drastic weight loss concerned her co-workers, and her skin took on a gray-tinged tone.

At her next appointment, her oncologist told her that he had an idea of what was causing her diarrhea. At that point, he became the first doctor to administer a test directly related to neuroendocrine tumor diagnosis; he ordered a 5HIAA test, a 24-hour test that measures serotonin metabolite levels in the urine. During that visit, he also mentioned to Marge that there was a medication available that he thought would help control the diarrhea, but that she would have to inject it daily. The thought of injecting medicine on a daily basis upset her, but at that point she would have done almost anything to stop the diarrhea. After her visit, she went to the lab for the urine test, and went home, feeling just as weak and nauseous as she had when she got there. By this time, she had lost her appetite, and was barely picking at her food. She was also thirsty, but nothing she drank seemed to quench her thirst. She spoke to my husband and he told her to drink some Gatorade. It was only in the emergency room later that she learned that she was suffering from severe hypokalemia, which is low blood potassium. This condition was brought on by the incessant diarrhea that Marge had been suffering from for over a month. The normal blood potassium level is 3.5 to 5. Marge's was 1.75. The on-call physician later told her that drinking Gatorade probably saved her life.

Two days later, Marge returned to the doctor to get the results of the urine tests. It was at that time that she was diagnosed with a VIPoma, (this diagnosis was revised later in treatment to a pancreatic carcinoid.) an extremely rare neuroendocrine tumor that produces profuse amounts of uncontrollable diarrhea. The clinic had been busy that day, and the wait had taken hours. By the time the doctor came into the room, Marge was nearly asleep in the examining room, her head on the desk. The doctor noted her discomfort, and her inability to walk, and quickly ordered blood tests. While she was relieved to actually have a diagnosis after years of battles, it didn't make her feel any better. At this point she could barely stay awake, and had fallen asleep at a stoplight on her way to the hospital clinic. When she went home, she simply passed out on the couch, unable to stay awake, and too weak to walk around.

When I talked to Marge the next day, I was alarmed. I could always tell by the tone of her voice how she felt. Her voice, normally bubbly and cheerful, would take on an almost sorrowful quality. Today, her voice was barely above a whisper. I urged her to talk to the doctor, and she promised that she would.

She never kept that promise.

The doctor called her instead.

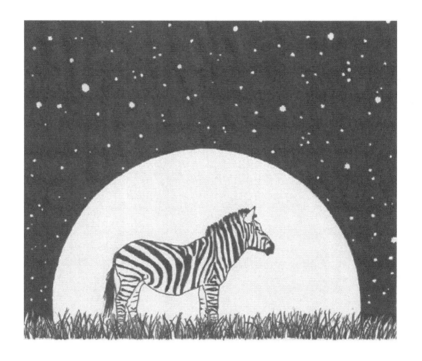

CHAPTER EIGHT
A Treatment of Sorts

"The next day was my dad's birthday. I had planned a birthday party to celebrate, but found myself collapsing after running some errands. I just lay on the couch, unable to move. My dad became concerned, and called my name often to see if I could respond. I was able to (barely), but I just couldn't find the strength to move. At 6:00 PM, the phone rang. My boyfriend Jesse helped me get to the phone. The caller was an associate of my doctor. She told me that my potassium was low, and that my doctor wanted me to come to the hospital ER. I asked her when, and she said 'right now.'

I asked her how low my potassium was. She said 1.75. I had no idea how dangerously low that was."

—From Marge's Diary

Low potassium would continue to plague my sister for the rest of her life. Not all carcinoid patients experience the drastic drop in potassium that Marge did. Although diarrhea is one of the most common symptoms of carcinoid syndrome, others experience a variety of symptoms, including pain, wheezing, flushing, and valvular heart disease. But this is why it is so important to receive an accurate, timely diagnosis. The sooner the symptoms of this disease are managed, the better quality of life carcinoid patients will experience. As mentioned earlier, the fallout from the symptoms are frequently what prove to be deadly, not the spread of the tumor itself.

Eventually, Marge ended up in the hospital for four days while she was given fifteen bags of potassium chloride in order to bring her potassium levels back to normal. When she was ready to leave the hospital, her legs were so swollen from the immense amounts of potassium she had received that it took nearly a week for them to return to normal size. It was also at this time that she began taking octreotide injections, which is specifically designed to inhibit the release of the hormones that flood the body, and can cause such harm.

She began taking 50 micrograms of octreotide a day. Her symptoms improved immediately, and her diarrhea lessened to a manageable level. But within three months her diarrhea had returned, and she began feeling tired again. The doctor increased her injection to 100 micrograms, which helped immediately. She maintained this dose from 1995 to 1999, when her diarrhea returned once more, along with another dangerous drop in potassium.

It didn't take long for Marge's potassium levels to get out of control. Her injections were increased to twice daily, and her doctor prescribed a potassium supplement for her to take twice a day. But by 2000, her symptoms again worsened. The doctor rewrote her prescription, adding a third injection. This seemed to help, and in fact, was the dose she stayed at for the next two years.

In the beginning of 2002, Marge's insurance informed her that her current doctor would no longer be a participating provider in her plan. It had taken her several years to get the correct diagnosis and a treatment plan that worked, and now she would have to begin all over again.

Marge eventually found a physician that was somewhat familiar with carcinoid. He ordered an extensive series of tests. But it was at this time that her diarrhea became particularly intense, and her doctor admitted that he was stumped. And because her potassium levels were dropping even quicker than before, she began making the trip to the clinic three times a week to have her potassium levels checked. On several occasions, she had to have a potassium IV in order to quickly get the levels back to normal.

She was also given a slew of new medications, which included an anti-diarrhea medication, additional potassium supplements, and a pancreatic enzyme. Her octreotide prescription was also increased to 300 micrograms, three times a day. Eventually her doctor placed her on pump infusion, but by that time, it did not do much to relieve her symptoms.

Through it all, whenever she was asked about her illness, there was always one sentence she would repeat, again and again.

"I am able to handle it."

These are such simple words, but they speak a great deal to the courage that Marge displayed throughout her bout with carcinoid cancer. She would frequently make jokes about her condition, particularly on bad days. When someone would ask her if she was okay, she would reply, " either it will pass or I will." Many people saw it as grim humor, but I saw it as a reflection of the person that she was; strong, courageous, and realistic. Humor got her through the hardest part of this disease, and even when she went into the hospital for the final time, she had packed away her hospital snacks in her suitcase to take home with her.

But they, like Marge, never made it home.

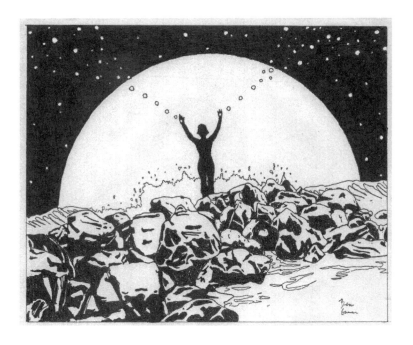

CHAPTER NINE
Living With Strength and Dignity

Although she stopped her personal journal in late 2002, I have many emails that I received from Marge that continued to show the type of person she was. And though her health began to take a downward spiral at this time, she continued to work full time. The last year of her life, she was on Total Parental Nutrition (TPN) because her body could no longer absorb nutrition from food. Three times a week, she had a potassium IV at home, along with the TPN, and any other nutrients that she needed. Quite a lot to pack for a vacation, but somehow she managed it.

That doesn't surprise me. For as long as I can remember, my sister was the tough one. I was the one that cried. As the 'little' sister, I was picked on. She would hit me and I would cry. Even when I learned that it would be better to hit back, I still cried. Until the day that I became tired of being the crybaby, and I bit her.

I can close my eyes and see that day so clearly in my mind, even though it was so very many years ago. Her face crumpled up, and she started to cry. I stared at her in horror. I don't think I had ever seen my sister cry. Not the way she did that day. Her shoulder sported a fresh bruise, courtesy of me.

I felt as awful as a five year old can feel. Not only did I hurt her, but I had also made her cry.

Even today, I can see her face crumpled up in pain.

That is the face that I continued to see throughout her twenty-year battle with this phantom disease called carcinoid cancer. No one else had privy to this face, but underneath her carefully made up face, I saw that same six-year-old girl crying out in pain. Marge was always careful about hiding her pain. Friends, co-workers and strangers only saw an attractive woman with blonde hair, bright green eyes, and stick straight posture. Some days she may have looked a little tired, or a little too pale, but don't we all at times?

I saw the little girl in pain. I was there during the rare times when she let her guard down, carefully removed her surface mask, and let her pain show.

As young girls, Marge was my closest friend, along with being the occasional disciplinarian. And although our fights continued, we both knew that we would always be there to help each other.

For so many years, Marge would refuse to talk about her illness. Even when she would come to visit me, she would warn me on the phone that she had lost some weight, and didn't want to talk about it. I respected her wishes, even when I could see that she was getting progressively sicker. Between 1998 and 1999, she lost a great deal of weight. Always a little heavy, her weight loss looked drastic and shocking, rather than healthy and attractive. Each visit, I held my breath as I waited for her at the airport, praying that she hadn't lost too much weight. My prayers were never answered. Every time I saw her, she was skinnier than she had been previously.

When she arrived to visit me in March of 2003, she looked thin and drawn. As she came closer, I felt a tremor of fear rush through me. She looked positively fragile, the veins in her hands raised prominently. Her upper arms were literally skin and bones, all traces of fat gone. I remembered her hands; they used to be slightly plump, as were her arms. Now her clothes hung off of her stick-thin frame, and her face looked drawn and pale. I didn't like it, but I also knew how upset she would be if I mentioned it. Marge never liked to be reminded of her illness, and although she wasn't in denial, she certainly disliked any mention of it at all. As a matter of fact, most of her friends and co-workers had no idea just how ill she was. My role in her life was to provide her with information about her disease that I had gathered from various websites, along with reassurance on those nights when her pain encompassed her whole being. Between reassurances, I offered her several alternatives to seeing her regular physician, including visits to various specialists. Although I promised I would make the calls and go along with her, she always listened, but continued to decline my advice.

During this vacation, Marge wanted us to drive to Las Vegas, and I agreed. The trip started out good, but midway between Albuquerque and Las Vegas, she began to feel ill. It soon became clear that things were not quite as 'good' as she had led me to believe.

The drive to Las Vegas in 2003 was very rough. As we drove through a winter storm in Flagstaff, AZ, I thought about what I could do to help her. We had to stop several times for Marge to use the bathroom. Her diarrhea was chronic and unstoppable, even with her medication.

Every time we had to stop, Marge kept saying, "I'm sorry." I knew she felt terrible, and so did I.

The rest of our vacation was relatively uneventful, but on our last night, she began having uncontrollable diarrhea again. Between Arizona and New Mexico, we had to make several stops, even on the side of the road, so she could vomit.

By the time we got home, we were both mentally and physically exhausted. I was upset that she would not let me share her pain and illness with her. She continued to shut me out. She was upset because I kept telling her to see another doctor, to take her retirement money and go see a carcinoid specialist. "What good does your retirement money do if you're not here to enjoy it?" I asked her, frustrated and angry.

She stayed curled up on my sofa, her pain apparent for everyone to see. Her anger at her illness caused her to spend the rest of the evening insulting me. The next day was no better, as we spent it snipping at each other non-stop; hers out of pain, mine out of frustration. That evening, my husband took me aside and said, "You two have to talk. You need to tell her that she needs to do something, or she'll die."

She'll die.

Words that both of us had studiously avoided. Words that I had refused to hear before but had no choice now but to acknowledge. I thought of Marge sitting on the sofa, stick thin, and ghostly white. I thought of her beautiful eyes, dull and unfocused as she tried to deal with her unrelenting pain. I thought of what my life would be without her.

It was midnight. Marge was sitting on the corner of the couch, curled up in a tiny ball. The room was dark.

I sat down next to her. "I'm sorry," I said, looking at her in the dark. "I know I've been a total bitch, but I'm so scared. You have to do something."

Silence.

"Take your money and go see someone, please," I said. "I'll go with you. What good is the money if you die? And you have to be around for Jared."

Jared is my son, and my sister was so incredibly proud of him. She adored him, and the feeling was mutual. Jared was my trump card, and I played it shamelessly.

"I know, I know. I'll call the doctor when I get home." She sounded weak and exhausted. And although I was happy to hear her finally agree, a part of me was frightened because she had. It was our first acknowledgement that she was ill, not just really ill, but terminally ill. And it frightened me.

"Please promise me you'll do something," I begged.

"I promise."

Marge went home the next day. Before we went to the airport, we stopped for breakfast, the first meal she was able to eat in two days. She looked a little better than she had, but was still drawn and weak. Later, when I left the airport, I tried to think positively, but for the first time, I couldn't shake the vision of Marge in the living room; thin, pale, and weak. And for the first time, I couldn't shake the feeling that things were going to get much, much worse.

When she got home, she did become much more aggressive in fighting her disease. After being hospitalized for stomach pain unrelated to her tumor, she had her gallbladder removed. There seemed to be an immediate improvement in her health after that. And when she visited Albuquerque in November, she looked better than she had in a while. Her pain, while still present, had subsided some, and to my amazement, she had even gained some weight.

On Saturday night, we went to the Native American Music Awards, a show that Marge and I had attended several times before. We ended up staying out all of Saturday night, and then stopped for breakfast on the way back to my house. It was so much like the way things used to be, it was almost painful.

When someone you love is ill, you try so hard to appreciate every single moment that you are together. Granted, it's nearly impossible to do this. We all end up getting impatient or aggravated about some thing that in retrospect seems unimportant. But that weekend, everything was perfect. When Marge got home she proudly told everyone that she had been so happy to be able to stay out late like she used to.

But our perfect weekend faded to December, when Marge started to get sick again. Her cycle always started the same; uncontrollable diarrhea followed by vomiting. Increased doses of octreotide did nothing to reduce the diarrhea. She quickly dropped fifteen pounds, and was hospitalized the week before Christmas.

I was planning on taking Jared and driving to Chicago after the holidays, only to come down with a bacterial infection in my throat, which quickly abscessed. Because it was contagious, I was told I would be unable to visit the hospital if indeed I made the drive to Chicago. By the time the abscess healed, Marge was released from the hospital on January 2, 2004.

It was during this last hospital stay that her doctor decided to prescribe TPN to help with her nutritional deficiency. She had continued to maintain the PICC line that the hospital had installed during her gallbladder surgery. The PICC was always used for the TPN and along with a

Potassium/Magnesium drip. This combination caused her legs to swell tremendously. She called me, miserable. Although her doctor told her that the TPN was not permanent, I felt another twinge as she described what her day entailed. And my admiration grew for her once again.

Three times a week, she was infused with TPN. On alternate days, she had a potassium and magnesium drip. Every morning before work, a home health nurse would come to the house, remove the lines, and clean them. My sister would then get dressed and head to work.

Just recently I'd had a bout with a nasty stomach virus. My family and I had been out for dinner and the evening had been terrific, when suddenly I developed severe stomach cramps. Within minutes, I knew that if I didn't find a restroom soon, I'd be in major trouble.

For the next twenty fours hours, I alternated between vomiting and having painful bouts of diarrhea. I was afraid to stray too far from the house for fear of an accident.

But the worst part was how bad I felt. I was weak and unstable. My head felt like it was floating in the clouds, and my legs felt like lead. All I wanted to do was lay down and go to sleep.

That evening, as I prepared for bed, something suddenly occurred to me.

How I felt today was exactly how Marge had felt every single day of her life during the last few years. Yet, somehow, she had managed to remain optimistic, even enthusiastic about life. She got up and went to work, and listened silently as her co-workers complained about their colds and various aches and pains. She went shopping, bought makeup, and got a manicure and a pedicure on a regular basis. She went on vacation, usually to visit me, or to her favorite place, Las Vegas.

Up until that day, I had absolutely no clue about what she had gone through on a regular basis. I knew my stomach virus didn't even come close compared to what my sister faced every day with strength, character, enthusiasm, and courage. I am so proud of her, of her incredible fight, of her determination, and of her ability to never, ever give up, even in the face of death.

There were many days when she felt like giving up, but she got dressed, albeit a little bit slower, put on her makeup, and drove herself ten miles to work each day.

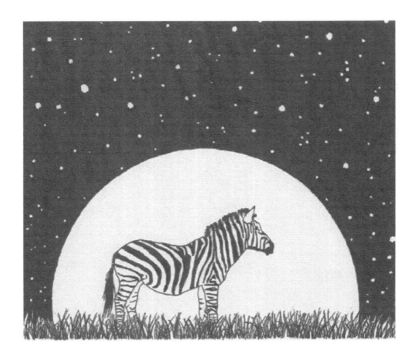

CHAPTER TEN
Spiritual Renewal

"Like the book says, 'let go and let God. I'm beginning to think this prayer stuff really works."

—*From Marge's Diary*

Marge and I were brought up Catholic. But in recent years, neither one of us was active in the Catholic Church. Although I felt sure that God existed, while growing up, I often questioned his presence. But I noticed that as Marge grew weaker, she began to turn to her faith, long forgotten. This seemed to provide her with additional strength, and she took comfort in prayer.

There were days when she called me depressed because her legs had swollen again, and it was hard to walk down the stairs. But then there were other days when we talked for hours about what color purse she should buy.

Here is just a sample of the emails I received from Marge several months before her death.

"I'm having a pity party today, and I don't know why. I do, but it's something that I have to work through on my own."

Marge refused to feel sorry for herself, and the last thing she wanted was pity from friends or co-workers. She took what was given to her in stride, and never looked back. She was at heart, a very private person, and never shared information about her carcinoid struggle with anyone but her closest friends.

"How's your day today? Good, I hope. Mine is okay, a little tired and still got the extra-large sausages. (Marge's legs swelled tremendously when she was on the TPN.) I talked to Cathy (her home nurse) this morning, and I'm trading in my PICC for a PORT. I'll tell you about it later."

Throughout all of her medical ordeals, Marge always kept her sense of humor. She always kept me updated about all of the medical procedures that she was having.

"Please tell Vicki I am grateful for all her prayer's and if she is rising in the middle of the night to pray for me, there is no doubt a miracle will soon follow."

One morning, when I went into work, my boss Vicki, who is also a very close friend, told me that she awoke at 2:00 AM with the sudden urge to pray for Marge. When I told Marge about this later, she started to cry, touched that someone that she knew only on a very casual basis, was praying for her.

"…my potassium went up to 3.2 (normal range is 3.5 to 5.0) and my mag (magnesium) was 2.0. I didn't know that if the magnesium is in the proper range, it helps keep the potassium levels normal. I have only had one 'blowout' since taking the opium. Who knows, maybe it does work. I am totally zoned."

When Marge began to experience more frequent diarrhea that was not controlled by her daily octreotide injections, her oncologist searched for an alternative. When he prescribed Tincture of Opium, Marge had reservations, but tried it anyway. It made her completely dysfunctional. Several times she found herself falling asleep at a stoplight on her way home from work. And this was from taking it the night before. Her system was very sensitive to narcotics, and while the Opium did slow down the diarrhea some, she was not able to do any of the things that she normally did. And a normal routine was extremely important to Marge. Keeping a normal schedule was her way of dealing with her illness. It was her way of keeping herself going, even on days when she should have never left her house.

"…I fell asleep in the chair last night. I think this may be part of the pain I have today in my legs and butt. I could barely walk; it took forever to get ready for work. I have 'Lincoln Logs' again (swollen legs). By the time I got to the car, all I could do was cry. This is one of those days when you want to 'chuck it all' but I talked to Dad (our Dad is deceased) and to God, and hopefully one of them was listening. I called Cindy (her friend) to vent, and it felt pretty good. I'm trying to think about the BIG LV (Las Vegas) and be positive, but there are just some days that are harder than others."

The constant infusion of TPN and potassium into her system caused Marge's legs to swell immensely. Although she had a diuretic prescribed, her doctor didn't want her to take it in case she lost more potassium. As a result, she often had a hard time moving around, particularly in the morning.

Marge and my dad were very close. She often visited the cemetery where he was buried to talk to him. A visit to the cemetery often gave her the strength to get through another day. And any talk of visiting Las Vegas was guaranteed to cheer her up. Marge loved Las Vegas. She was content just being there, playing slot machines, walking down the Strip, or sitting outside, watching the sunrise over the mountains. If anyone ever asked Marge where she wanted to go, the answer was always "Las Vegas."

"...I'm sure you noticed the subject line is 'I'm Nervous.' This is the first time since seeing Dr.*** that I feel totally anxious. Maybe because there is a chance that they are taking away everything I've come to rely on. I was so sick here at work yesterday that three people asked if I needed help in the bathroom. I was crouched down on the floor. BILE will do that to a person. My appointment is at 5:40. I'll call you as soon as I get home, maybe on the way home."

This email came shortly after her oncologist told her that he was taking her off both octreotide and TPN. His theory was that perhaps the injections were making her worse, not better. So he told her the week before that on her next visit, he would be stopping both, "just to see what happened."

Unfortunately, stopping the octreotide injections had the expected results. She was sicker, if that was possible, than she had been before. Within days, he put her back on the injections, but the brief lapse had taken its toll. She spent nearly a week in the hospital hooked up to numerous IV's in order to replace all of the vital fluids that she lost during those few days. It took her nearly a month to recover from that ill advised medical decision.

"I think I'm gonna be okayyyyyyyyyyy! When I got up this morning, things looked much brighter. I even picked out the majority of the stuff I'm taking with. VIVA LAS VEGAS!!!!"

This email came just days before our trip to Las Vegas. But as she was happily planning on what clothes to wear, her port, which had been inserted in February, became infected. She ended up at the hospital on Sunday with a fever of 101.5. She was due to fly from Chicago to Las Vegas on Thursday. On Tuesday, after her fever came down, the port was removed and the PICC line reinserted. And on Thursday, she was on a plane, headed to Las Vegas.

In June 2004, Marge visited Albuquerque for what turned out to be the last time. We had celebrated her birthday in May in Las Vegas, but we had never had a birthday cake. So for her visit, I brought a birthday cake for her. She was surprised and pleased. During her visit, we had birthday cake and coffee for breakfast each day. On Friday, we went to a concert featuring Jim Boyd, one of her favorite musicians. Marge had always wanted to meet him, but was too shy to say so. I was able to finally introduce them, and she went home ecstatic that she had been able to finally meet and speak to him. Of course the trip ended up taking its toll on her, and she spent the next few days in the hospital. Within days she was back to work.

"...I'm here, (at work) movin' slower than a snail and as big as a house, but I'm here. My potassium was 3.4 yesterday, so I guess taking the extra bag (of potassium) must have helped."

Jared and I visited Marge in Chicago in July. She had just had a chemoembolization (her first) in June, and was still recovering. But instead of the usual symptoms present after a chemoembolization, her major symptom was abdominal swelling. She was discouraged because several people had asked her if she was pregnant. A subsequent visit to the doctor assured her that the swelling was normal and that it should begin to recede shortly. Because she had spent so much time at the hospital, she felt she was unable to take any time off while Jared and I were there. Unfortunately, we didn't get to spend much time together. The day that Jared and I left, we hugged goodbye in the living room. On the morning we were leaving, I woke up early to say goodbye to her. I was still tired, but here she was, dressed and looking incredibly pretty, if a little tired. I hugged her tight, and watched as she hugged my son. It never occurred to me that that would be the last time I would see her, hug her, kiss her. I wouldn't have let her go quite so easy.

After Marge left for work, Jared and I went to breakfast with Jesse. As we sat in the small, neighborhood diner, I remembered back a few years, when I had visited Chicago alone. Marge and I had sat in this same restaurant, on a cold, rainy day, drinking coffee for hours. We spent hours talking, as rain misted the windows. After about two hours, she looked at me and said, "Do you know how long I've been wanting to do this?"

I had no idea. We often kidded each other about moving closer to one another. I wanted her to come to New Mexico, and she wanted me to come back to Chicago. We both had jobs we enjoyed, and I had the additional responsibility of my son. As a result, we were never able to come to terms with where we should be. But distance didn't keep us apart. Marge visited New Mexico two or three times a year, and I usually made it to Chicago at least once or twice a year. And over the years the distance between us made each of us appreciate the other more. As a result, we fought less, and were able to enjoy our time together.

But as Jesse, Jared, and I sat at the restaurant, I couldn't seem to shake this empty feeling inside of me. So much had changed since that day five years ago. Marge had gotten progressively sicker, and as much as she tried to deny it, nothing seemed to be helping her.

Suddenly, I didn't want to be there. It seemed so wrong that she wasn't there. It was more than just missing a person for a moment. It was more of a reality check; what the world would be like when Marge was gone. Everything was the same, but yet different. It just wasn't right. And it hasn't been since the day Marge decided she had enough and moved on to a better place.

CHAPTER ELEVEN
The Life of a Cancer Cell

"All cancer cells begin life the same way," says Dr. Eugene Woltering, Chief, Section Endocrine Surgery and the James D. Rives Professor of Surgery, and Chief, Section of Surgical Endocrinology, Department of Surgery, Louisiana State University Medical Center in New Orleans. He illustrates his point by putting a single pencil dot on a pad of legal paper. This single dot, Dr. Woltering explains, is one cancer cell. When this cell eventually divides, it becomes two cells. When those two cells divide again, there will be four cancer cells.

"The time it takes for the cells to split and divide is called the doubling time," says Dr. Woltering. "Because every tumor, like a fingerprint, is unique, every tumor has its own doubling time. The longer the doubling time, the happier the patient is, because they live longer."

"For instance," Dr. Woltering continues, "let's use 180 days as doubling time. In other words, 180 days is the time it will take for one cancer cell to become two cancer cells. In another 180 days, those two cancer cells will become four cancer cells. In another 180 days, those four cancer cells will become eight cancer cells. When a cancer cell is this small, it is virtually undetectable in your body. The common wisdom is that it usually takes ten, twelve, even fifteen doubling times before a tumor can be detected at all. That applies to all types of cancer, found in any part of the body."

Unless invasive action is taken, (surgical removal, chemotherapy, etc.) the tumor will continue to grow at this rate. According to Dr. Woltering, doubling times vary widely, so for traditionally slow growing cancers like carcinoid, it can take a very long time to reach the size of a pencil eraser. And once it reaches the size of a pencil eraser, growth will appear to become faster, even though it isn't. It's just that there is more tumor mass now doubling. That is why, Dr. Woltering explains, that as you get closer to the end of your life, it appears as if the tumor growth is more rapid, but it's essentially the mathematics. In Dr. Woltering's words, "the mathematics screw you."

So the solution is to get diagnosed as soon as possible. But how do you do that when the symptoms of carcinoid are so similar to those of many other diseases? What are the best tests to ask your doctor to perform? And what do the results of those tests tell you?

CHAPTER TWELVE
Do I Have A Carcinoid Tumor?

Many carcinoid patients are incredibly well versed in the diagnosis and treatment of their disease, having had no choice but to become proactive in order to obtain the proper treatment. As information becomes more easily accessible, health care workers, including physicians, are becoming much more knowledgeable about carcinoid cancer. Hopefully there will come a time when patients can expend their energies on something other than convincing another physician that they need treatment.

Health professionals often encourage their patients to play a more proactive role in their health management and treatment options. But because of the relative rarity of carcinoid tumors, carcinoid patients are often forced to become very knowledgeable very quickly. It's not unusual for a doctor to see only one or two carcinoid patients throughout their entire career, if they see one at all.

The lack of consistent treatment protocol is one of the reasons why Dr. Eugene Woltering M.D., believes that instead of the doctor educating the doctor, when treating carcinoid patients, it's better to educate the patient, who in turn can educate their own doctor.

"Say you're a medical oncologist who sees a thousand patients a year," says Dr. Woltering. "Nine hundred and ninety nine of those patients have common cancers such as lung, breast, or colon. You may have one carcinoid patient. So when it's time to attend a conference, which one do you attend; the one that teaches you how to treat the nine hundred and ninety nine, or the one that teaches you how to treat a single carcinoid patient?"

That is one of the main reasons why the annual Carcinoid Conference was created. Since 1997, an annual conference has taken place, held in various locations throughout the U.S. Carcinoid experts from across the country (and world) are brought in to discuss the various aspects of the disease, discuss current research projects and talk about the latest treatment protocols. What sets these conferences apart from the typical medical conference is that carcinoid patients and caregivers are part of the conference as well.

"That's what these (conferences) are all about," says Dr. Woltering. "Arming the patients with a pile of literature authored by carcinoid experts to take back to their own physicians."

According to Dr. Woltering this approach works well. "Sure, you'll run into the occasional curmudgeon who, if you told him you had the cure for cancer, would simply tell you to take a hike," Dr. Woltering admits. "But for the most part, the doctors are very receptive to this approach."

The carcinoid conference continues to grow. In the last three years, attendance averaged 350 patients and caregivers. In 2005, attendees came from 36 states, and from as far away as Great Britain.

Carcinoid is a deeply individual disease. That is what makes this disease particularly frustrating for those who treat carcinoid patients on a regular basis.

"If I see fourteen people with this disease, I've seen fourteen different complexities," says Dr. Lowell Anthony. But Dr. Anthony goes on to note that there are also similarities, which typically can include flushing, diarrhea, wheezing, and fatigue.

But just how easy is it to diagnose carcinoid or neuroendocrine tumors? The rarity of their occurrence means that many physicians are just not looking for them. There are approximately 8,000 cases of carcinoid tumors diagnosed in the United States each year. Some of these patients are diagnosed during routine surgery for an unrelated illness or injury. Others are diagnosed because of related illnesses such as unexplained intestinal bleeding or bowel obstruction. Still others complain of vague symptoms such as nausea, undiagnosed pain, and flushing for years before receiving an accurate diagnosis.

And while these symptoms can certainly signal carcinoid, they frequently point to much more common diseases. The vagueness of these symptoms also illustrates the problem with diagnosing carcinoid early. And because of the relative rareness of carcinoid and neuroendocrine tumors in general, testing for these tumors is usually last on the list, if it makes the list at all.

It's common knowledge that if cancer is diagnosed early it can often mean the difference between long-term survival or even remission, and a premature death. The same is true for carcinoid patients. Unfortunately, a carcinoid diagnosis does not guarantee that a proper treatment protocol will be implemented. In fact, a carcinoid diagnosis often leads to confusion resulting in the delay of proper treatment.

By far, the most common approach when treating a newly diagnosed carcinoid patient is the 'wait and see' approach. Used in cases where the tumor is discovered during unrelated surgery or other testing, the doctor will usually employ this type of treatment when symptoms are relatively mild, and not disruptive to the patient's quality of life. Because of the slow growth of these tumors, doctors are often not comfortable recommending surgery, or other aggressive treatments when the patient is relatively symptom free. This approach can work well for years providing that the patient's tumors, blood and urine are monitored on a regular basis, and checked for any signs of change The doctor's opinion is that once activity is discovered, a more aggressive treatment will be prescribed. The biggest drawback to this approach is that once carcinoid metastasizes to other sites, particularly the liver, it becomes much more difficult to contain, and the symptoms become harder to keep under control.

"Our group feels that you should make an aggressive search for the primary (tumor) and remove it. If it can't be removed, resect it," says Dr. Woltering. "The primary is like a dandelion. If it remains in the body, you'll be seeding more cells into circulation."

In fact, carcinoid specialists tend to agree that if the primary tumor is found and removed, the patient stands a good chance of being cured.

Many physicians see this aggressive approach as unnecessary, and even risky. And obviously, there is always some risk when surgery is involved, particularly major surgery. But an aggressive approach at the beginning may eliminate the need for more risky procedures later down the road.

"Either an aggressive or a non-aggressive approach is okay if you monitor markers every three months, and do scans every six months," says Dr. Woltering, "but if you get three to six months behind the eight-ball, you can get in deep trouble."

CHAPTER THIRTEEN
Testing and Treatment

If your physician suspects a carcinoid tumor, he or she will probably order the following tests. Additional testing of various hormones can also be undertaken if a diagnosis remains uncertain.

CHROMOGRANIN A (CgA) TESTING

Studies have estimated that CgA blood levels are elevated in at least 80 percent of Carcinoid patients, making this one of the best diagnostic tests to order if carcinoid is suspected. Granin is a protein found in granules inside neuroendocrine cells and is typically produced by both carcinoid and other neuroendocrine tumors. Measuring the CgA levels can indicate to physicians the amount of tumor that is present in the body. Normally, the higher the CgA levels, the more tumor load the patient has.

5-HIAA

Along with the CgA, this is usually one of the first tests that are given once Carcinoid is suspected. 5-HIAA (5-hydroxy indole acetic acid) measures the level of serotonin by-products in the urine over a 24-hour period. Those with a functioning carcinoid tumor will almost always have an elevated level of 5-HIAA. There are several foods that must be avoided for 24 to 48 hours prior to taking the test because they can produce an inaccurately raised level. Those foods include bananas, pineapples, avocados, walnuts, caffeine, and Tylenol, along with a host of other medications.

Along with Chromogranin-A and 5-HIAA, other tests to screen for possible carcinoid include Serotonin, Pancreastatin, Neurokinen-A, and Substance-P level testing.

Another important test to consider is the Ki-67. This is done using sample tissue taken during a biopsy of a tumor, and is done to determine the number of cells currently undergoing mitosis, which is the process of cell division. When this is completed, a grade is assigned to the tumor(s), and used to determine disease progression. The lower the Ki-67 number is, the better. This is an important test, and should be done on all patients who have been diagnosed with a carcinoid, or other neuroendocrine tumor.

LOCATING TUMORS

Various methods can be used to locate the site of the primary tumor, and to detect any tumor spread. CT (Computed Tomography) and MRI (Magnetic Resonance Imaging) scans are often used to detect the presence of tumors in the body. These scans can normally show the location of tumors. An Octreotide scan is where a radioactive agent is combined with octreotide and injected into the patient's vein. The octreotide will bind to the receptors that are normally found on carcinoid cell membranes. A nuclear camera enables radiologists to locate and display the areas where these tumors are found.

I-123 and I-131 MIBG scans can also be used to improve diagnostic accuracy. These are radiolabeled scans that use meta-iodobenzylguanidine instead of octreotide, to bind to tumor receptors.

IF A TUMOR IS FOUND

If a tumor is located and removed, or a biopsy obtained, a special staining test for Chromogranin A should be completed. This test can determine the degree of differentiation of the tumor. Differentiation is used to determine cancer progression. A well-differentiated cell resembles the normal tissue that it derived from and is considered a low-grade cancer. A poorly differentiated c looks more primitive and is considered a high-grade cancer. The higher the percent of cells that stain positive for CgA, the better the outlook is.

SOME TREATMENTS FOR CARCINOID CANCER

Below you will find common treatments used for patients diagnosed with carcinoid and other neuroendocrine tumors. The list is by no means a treatment recommendation, nor is it a complete list of treatment options.

SURGERY

Surgery is by far the best treatment for carcinoid cancer patients. Even though surgery is frequently avoided by physicians because of inherent risk factors, surgery is the only treatment that may provide a complete cure of carcinoid cancer, provided the tumor is removed before it has spread to other organs. Even patients with metastases can benefit from surgery. Reducing tumor mass can also reduce symptoms, since debulking the tumor can reduce the amount of hormones released into the bloodstream.

Although any type of surgery carries a risk, surgery on carcinoid tumors presents an additional risk: Carcinoid Crisis. Carcinoid crisis can occur during surgery, causing either a spike in blood pressure (hypertensive crisis) or a sudden drop in blood pressure (hypotensive crisis). Neither of these can be predicted prior to surgery, and carcinoid specialists commonly concur that octreotide be used or available during any surgical procedure.

BIOTHERAPY

There are currently three types of somatostatin analogs available worldwide. Octreotide (which is the only one of the three available in the United States), Lanreotide, and

Vapreotide.   All three of these drugs can be injected subcutaneously, intra-muscularly, (which provides a slow-release of the drug,) or intravenously. In the U.S., Octreotide is the accepted treatment for carcinoid and other neuroendocrine tumors.

CHEMOEMBOLIZATION

Because of the unique design of the liver, a procedure like chemoembolization is possible. Via a catheter inserted into the groin, chemotherapy drugs and embolizing particles are injected directly into the hepatic artery, which carries the blood supply that feeds liver tumors. A stronger chemotherapy agent is typically used, since the drugs remain in the liver and do not spread throughout the body. This also reduces the level of side effects that patients may suffer, which can include nausea, vomiting, and hair loss. And since the particles injected keep the drugs from spreading through the body, they are kept in close contact with the tumor, thus providing more effective treatment.

Chemoembolization is not without risks. As many as five in 100 patients die from complications directly related to chemoembolization. Risks can include liver infection and liver failure. Chemoembolization has been shown to extend the life of patients with liver tumors by about five years (average) but it is important to have this procedure done by an experienced interventional radiologist.

RADIOFREQUENCY ABLATION

Radiofrequency Ablation uses radiofrequency heat to burn cancer cells. This is done by inserting a needle directly into the tumor. The needle contains several prongs that are extended into the tumor. These prongs are able to deliver the radiofrequency heat directly into the tumor, burning the cancerous cells. Another procedure, called Cryoblation, is able to freeze the tumors and kill the cancer cells. This procedure is commonly recommended for smaller tumors.

HIGH DOSE INDIUM-111 PENTETREOTIDE THERAPY

Recently approved by the FDA for experimental protocol directed therapy in the U.S., this treatment is available for patients who have not responded to chemotherapy or radiation therapy. This is a tumor-targeted therapy that combines somatostatin analogs with radioactive Indium. The treatment is given by intravenous infusion over a period of several hours.

CLINICAL STUDIES

Clinical studies frequently take place in various locations across the United States. To search for clinical studies for carcinoid or neuroendocrine tumors, please visit www.ClinicalTrials.org. This website allows you to obtain in-depth information about clinical trials, search for trials by disease or location, and find out what the study requirements are. Clinical Trials can also be contacted by telephone at 888-FINDNLM (346-3656).

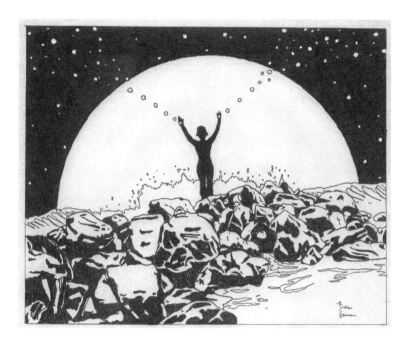

CHAPTER FOURTEEN
Finally Home

May 8th, 2005.

Today is Marge's birthday and also the day that we are here in Las Vegas to do what she had asked me to do; spread her ashes at the Stardust. It seems odd to be here without Marge. I walk past the eye-jolting maze of slot machines sitting at odd angles. At each turn, I expect to see her at one of the machines, straight-backed, blonde hair in a ponytail, playing a slot machine. As I walk mindlessly through the casino, I begin to think about what has happened in the last year. I quickly revise my original thought.

Marge is here.

She is here, at every restaurant we have ever eaten at. She is at the theater where we saw Wayne Newton. She is at the bar, drinking a cup of coffee in a small glass, with a napkin held in place by a rubber band. She is in the gift shop, buying a long sleeved shirt because the casino air conditioning was making her cold. She is at the slot machines, watching intently as the reels spin around and around. I may not be able to see her, but she is here.

I go outside to get some fresh air, and I feel her beside me, as we silently watch the water bounce from fountain to fountain. This was our refuge; this was our home away from home. The Stardust was Marge's favorite place in the world, and now she will be here for eternity. I go back inside convinced that if Marge's spirit is anywhere, it is here, at the Stardust.

Later that night, we all meet to discuss spreading her ashes. I haven't mentioned our plans to any Stardust employees or managers. They may not consider our plan a good marketing strategy.

In keeping with Marge's sense of humor, we divide her ashes amongst us, putting them in the Stardust's plastic coin cups. I hope she is watching us do this. I'm pretty sure that if she is, she's laughing pretty hard right now.

It's dark out when we finally decide that it's time to put Marge where she belongs. We all split up, taking our cups with us. My husband Shannon takes our son Jared, because this is something I need to do alone.

I remember when my Dad died. Shannon and I flew to Chicago to help arrange the funeral. I remember sitting at the table in the funeral home next to Marge, as we made painful decisions such as what kind of casket to buy, service times, funeral times, and obituary wording. I also remember thinking how grateful I was that Marge was there, sitting next to me. Just her presence made dealing with my father's death a little easier.

When my family and I arrived in Chicago after Marge's death, I somehow kept expecting her to be there, to make things better. When we arrived at the same funeral home, to make many of the same decisions that she and I had made eight years earlier, I struggled to suppress the panic that threatened to rise in me. Where was Marge? Why isn't she here with me? I can't do this alone. I can't.

I did.

My rational mind knew that Marge was not there; would never be there again. I would need to deal with that, starting right now. But as we made inane choices such as what newspapers to put her obituary in, I felt the panic threaten to rise again. After all, hadn't Marge always been there?

Not this time.

Not anymore.

'Did you think she was going to be here to help with her own funeral?' I berated myself.

No, I didn't think that. I didn't think we should be here at all. Marge wasn't supposed to die. She was only 48.

She had so many things left to accomplish. She had so many places left to visit.

But it wasn't up to me. It was Marge's time to go. That meant no more calls to Marge in the morning after I dropped my son off at school. No more waiting for her at the airport in Albuquerque when she would come to visit. The Kokopelli blanket she wanted for Christmas would remain in the store, or be bought by someone else. No more Christmas morning calls, talking about old traditions, new ones that we were trying to establish, and the hope that one year, we could spend Christmas together again. She would not be here to see my son grow up. I would no longer get a phone call asking me what purse she should buy, or what color lipstick would go with her new shirt, or if she should highlight her hair.

I might be wrong. Maybe Marge did stay around to help, because somehow I found an inner strength that I didn't know I had.

That was nine months ago. A lifetime ago. Now it was May, the month that we always visited Las Vegas. May was her favorite time to be in her favorite place in the world.

Tonight was the grand finale. I was hoping for a little more of that inner strength one more time. Because tonight was the official goodbye.

I went to a remote part of the Stardust, behind the pool and near the spa. It's a beautiful area with palm trees, sweet jasmine, and honeysuckle nearby. Before I tipped the cup, I looked out at the place where we had spent so many days and nights just having fun. I looked at the place that she loved so much, knowing that, like the restaurant in Chicago, it would never be the same again.

"You know, things just aren't the same here without you," I whispered into the darkness. It was true. Some days, I still felt so lost without her. I wondered if that feeling would ever go away. A part of me was missing without her. I knew that time would continue to shrink the giant hole that her death had left inside me. I knew that I would grow more comfortable with the emptiness, and on some days, not even notice it. But I also knew that it would never be replaced or filled by anything, or anyone else.

"You're getting want you wanted." I said, looking at the plastic Stardust coin cup in my hand. I thought briefly about what someone would think if they saw me now: a woman in her forties, alone, standing next to a palm tree, talking to a plastic cup.

"You could have just moved here, you know." I started to laugh out loud, and then quickly quieted myself. Was I losing it? I didn't know, and I didn't really care.

I continued along the small path until I was behind the palm trees. It felt like the perfect place. As I began to tip the cup to spread the ashes, a sudden gust of wind appeared. Instead of physically tipping the cup to spread the ashes, they were now just leaving the cup of their own accord, flowing effortlessly into the wind. I watched as they swirled in front of me, the cup still only partially tipped.

I smiled. Apparently Marge approved of the spot I chose.

When the cup was empty, I returned to the lit path, only to have my mouth drop in amazement. I watched silently from the sidewalk as Marge's ashes danced in front of me, swirling faster and faster until they resembled a miniature tornado. For a moment I wished someone were with me, to witness this. But I shook my head. I was glad I was alone. I felt that this was one last time for Marge and I to be at the Stardust together, just the two of us. Her ashes swirled faster. I watched as they lifted towards the heavens.

I looked at the area behind the lights where the ashes had been swirling. It was totally clear. I smiled to myself, feeling better than I had in a long time. I had witnessed something beautiful and miraculous, something that I wouldn't forget for a long time.

I headed back inside the casino to meet with the others. When I got to their table, my friend lightly touched me on the cheek.

"Ashes," she said as I looked at her questioningly. "That was Marge, giving you a kiss goodbye."

"She was thanking you for doing what she asked," said my husband.

After what I had witnessed earlier, I have no doubt that both my friend and my husband were correct. At that moment, I knew that Marge had been there beside me, and that she would continue to be beside me when I needed her most.

I smiled as I put my hand to my cheek and touched the ashes. At that moment, I was convinced that Marge was still here.

And she always would be.

Forever.

Resources

If you or a loved one has been recently diagnosed with carcinoid, or your physician suspects you have carcinoid, where can you find help, additional information, and access to carcinoid support groups around the world?

First and foremost, contact The Carcinoid Cancer Foundation. Founded in 1968, the Carcinoid Cancer Foundation's mission is "to encourage and support research and to educate the general public and health care professionals regarding carcinoid and related neuroendocrine tumors."

The foundation's website, www.carcinoid.org, contains informational resources for both patients and physicians. You can also find transcripts from conferences, medical information, links to support groups and a complete list of physicians who are currently considered the top specialists in the world. The foundation's goal is to encourage and conduct research, provide grants to various projects and support groups, provide up-to-date information on carcinoid and neuroendocrine tumors, and provide educational materials for both patients and their caregivers, along with medical professionals. Here you can also find extensive information on the latest treatments and clinical trials. The medical director of the Carcinoid Cancer Foundation is Dr. Richard R.P. Warner, a pioneer for carcinoid research and treatment, having spent nearly forty years researching and treating this disease.

When visiting the Carcinoid Foundation's website; (www.carcinoid.org), you will also find links to U.S. support groups in 29 states, along with links to support groups in Australia, Canada, Germany, The Netherlands, Norway, Sweden, and the United Kingdom.

Another source of information is The Caring For Carcinoid Foundation. Founded by Nancy and Patrick

O'Hagen in December 2004, the mission of The Caring For Carcinoid Foundation is to find a cure for carcinoid cancer in the next 7 to 10 years. 100 percent of the donations received by The Caring For Carcinoid Foundation are earmarked toward research for finding a cure. Their website, www.caringforcarcinoid.org features detailed information on various research projects that are in progress, along with a list of their Board of Scientific Advisors.

While both of these foundations are very different, they are alike in one very important way: both are dedicating every resource they can to finding a cure for carcinoid cancer.

OTHER RESOURCES

There are a variety of additional resources available to those who have been diagnosed with carcinoid or other neuroendocrine tumors. Those resources are listed below.

The Carcinoid Cancer Online Support Group is sponsored by the Association of Cancer Online Resources (ACOR). To join the list, go to listserv@listserve.acor.org. There are currently over 500 active members, which include patients with a current diagnosis of carcinoid, as well as caregivers.

Carcinoid@yahoogroups.com is an informational e-list. This is not a support group, but provides information about carcinoid tumors.

http://ca.groups.yahoo.com/group/carcinoidnetcanada/ This is a Canadian carcinoid support group.

There are also several websites that provide excellent information to both patients and caregivers. Many sites also provide valuable medical information for physicians and other healthcare personnel.

www.carcinoid.org/uk
This is the Hammersmith Hospital Carcinoid and
Neuroendocrine Tumor Service homepage. This site
contains information on current research programs, testing
information, and metabolic studies.

www.endotext.com
Endotex.com has an excellent section written primarily by
Dr. Aaron Vinik, an Eastern Virginia Medical School
Professor and Vice Chairman for Research. Titled "Diffuse
Hormonal Systems and Endocrine Tumor Syndromes," it
contains detailed information on a variety of neuroendocrine
tumors.

http://research.dfci.harvard.edu/neurocendocrine/index.php
This site contains excellent information on carcinoid and
related neuroendocrine tumors. Also available are detailed
facts on both localized and metastatic carcinoid disease,
including current treatment options.

www.pubmedcentral.nih.gov
This site contains a free archive where you can search for
carcinoid or other neuroendocrine tumor related articles. Use
'Carcinoid' as the keyword for your search.

www.carcinoid.com
Contains valuable information about carcinoid syndrome and
treatment options. The site is sponsored by Novartis, the
drug company that manufactures Sandostatin LAR®, an
injectable suspension of Octreotide Acetate, and currently the
gold standard for first line treatment to control the symptoms
of carcinoid syndrome.

www.nettumoradvisor.org
This website is dedicated to all types of neuroendocrine
tumors and takes you through symptoms, diagnosis,
treatment, monitoring, and current research data.

Carcinoid Specialists

Here is a list of doctors who have known experience in diagnosing and treating carcinoid and other neuroendocrine tumors. This is list is not meant to be exclusive, rather, it is meant to highlight those who have documented experience in treating Carcinoid. For a more complete listing, please refer to www.carcinoid.org. The listing is in alphabetical order, it is not exhaustive, and is not meant to be an endorsement of any or all of the physicians mentioned.

Jaffer A. Ajani
M.D. Anderson Cancer Center
1515 Holcombe Blvd.
Houston, TX 77030
713-792-2828
713-745-1163

Lowell Anthony M.D.
www.medschool.lsuhsc.edu
lantho@lsuhsc.edu
Kenner Regional Medical Center Office Building
200 W. Esplanade Ave.
Kenner, LA 70065
504-712-8701
504-465-2127 (fax)

Anthony P. Heaney M.D. PhD
Cedars Sinai Medical Center
The Carcinoid and Neuroendocrine Tumor Center
www.csmc.edu
8700 Beverly Blvd.
Suite 131
800-233-2771

310-423-4774
310-423-0440

David P. Kelsen M.D.
Memorial Sloan Kettering Cancer Center
1275 York Avenue
New York, NY 10021
646-497-9053 (New Patients)
212-639-8470

Matthew Kulke M.D.
Dana Farber Cancer Institute
www.dfci.harvard.edu
matthew_kulke@dfci.harvard.edu
44 Binney St.
Dana 1220
Boston, MA 02115
617-632-5136

Larry K. Kvols M.D.
Moffitt Cancer Center and Research Institute
www.moffitt.usf.edu
canceranswers@moffitt.usf.edu
12909 Magnolia Dr.
Tampa, FL 33612
813-903-3519

Irvin M. Modlin M.D. PhD
www.yalesurgery.med.yale.edu
Irvin.modlin@yale.edu
Yale School of Medicine
P.O. Box 208026
New Haven, CN 06520
203-785-5429
203-737-4067 (fax)

Jeffrey A. Norton M.D.

Stanford Comprehensive Cancer Center
300 Pasteur Drive
Stanford, CA   94305
650-7235461
650-736-1663
janorton@stanford.edu

Thomas O'Dorosio M.D.
University of Iowa Healthcare
www.uihealthcare.com
Thomas-odorisio@uiowa.edu
200 Hawkins Dr.
Iowa City, IA 52242
319-356-8133
319-356-4200

Rodney F. Pommier M.D.
Oregon Health Sciences University
www.oshu.edu
3181 S.W. Sam Jackson Park Road
Portland, OR 97239
503-494-5501

Joseph Rubin M.D.
Mayo Clinic Cancer Center
www.mayo.edu
222 First St. SW
Rochester, MN 55905
For appointment or more information
 call 507-538-3270

Leonard Saltz M.D.
Memorial Sloan-Kettering Cancer Center
1275 York Ave.
New York, NY 10021
646-497-9053 (New Patients)
212-639-21501

Alan P. Venook M.D.
venook@cc.ucsf.edu
P.O. Box 1705 UCSF
San Francisco, CA 94143-1705
415-353-9888
415-353-9959 (fax)
617-632-5370 (fax)

Aaron I. Vinik M.D. PhD
Eastern Virginia Medical School
vinikai@evms.edu
Diabetes Institutes South Campus
855 W. Brambleton Ave.
Norfolk, VA 23510
757-446-5912
757-446-5975 (fax)

Richard R.P. Warner M.D.
Medical Director – Carcinoid Cancer Foundation
1751 York Avenue
New York, NY 10128
212-722-2100 or 212-831-3031
www.carcinoid.org

Edward M. Wolin M.D.
Cedars-Sinai Comprehensive Care Center
8700 Beverly Blvd.
Los Angeles, CA 90048
310-423-0709
310-657-0737 (fax)

Eugene A. Woltering M.D.
www.medschool.lsuhsc.edu
ewolte@lsuhsc.edu
Kenner Regional Medical Center Office Building
200 W. Esplanade Ave.

Kenner, LA 70065
504-712-8701
504-45-2127(fax)

Dr. James C. Yao
M.D. Anderson Cancer Center
1515 Holcombe Blvd.
Houston, TX 77030
713-792-2828
713-745-1163

New Treatments On The Horizon

On October 25th, 1988, the Food and Drug Administration approved octreotide acetate (Sandostatin® for treatment of the chronic and debilitating diarrhea commonly associated with carcinoid and other neuroendocrine tumors. Prior to the availability of Sandostatin®, patients were frequently left weak from chronic diarrhea, and were often hospitalized for vital fluid replacement. According to Dr. Anthony, common treatments for those diagnosed with carcinoid tumors during the 1960's and 1970's included steroids and opiates such as Tincture of Opium and Paregoric. During this time period, says Dr. Anthony, median survival averaged around two years. After octreotide was approved in the U.S. for use on carcinoid patients, the period from 1985 through 1995 saw median survival rates climb to just over ten years. From 1996 through the current time frame, thanks to the use of octreotide acetate in its long lasting formulation (Sandostatin LAR®), median survival rates have now reached just over 16 years. Dr. Anthony estimated that the average person diagnosed with carcinoid lives approximately twenty years. This timeframe depends heavily on the primary tumor site, how advanced the disease is when it is discovered, and if the primary tumor has been removed. It's frustrating getting an accurate diagnosis, but Dr. Anthony stresses that it is important that you do not give up until you receive the correct diagnosis, and the correct treatment.

The creation of the North American Association of Patients With Neuroendocrine Tumors (NAPPNETS) has been an exciting development. Spearheaded by Dr. Woltering, the purpose of NAAPNETS is to offer a combined resource center for both carcinoid and other neuroendocrine tumor patients. This fusing of resources will also offer them a great deal more political clout.

The Caring For Carcinoid Foundation is optimistic about the future as well. Because they devote 100 percent of their donations directly to research, they estimate that they should be able to discover a cure for carcinoid in 7 to 10 years. Their concentration is on the genetics of cancer. The Caring For Carcinoid Foudantion references researchers who state that if they can determine what causes normal cells to mutate and cause carcinoid, they can develop targeted therapies that can stop, or deactivate those same mutations.

Carcinoid patients today have more treatment options than ever before. Some of the newest treatments involve radiolabeled somatostatin analogs. If tumors have receptors for somatostatin, which can be determined by an octreoscan, radiolabled isotopes such as Indium, Yttrium, In-Pentetreotide, or Rhenium can be attached to the somatostatin analog (octreotide) and delivered directly to the tumor receptors. Cytotoxic analogs of somatostatin are also being tested. Anti-angiogenic agents are one of the most exciting developments according to Dr. Woltering. "Tumors can't grow without blood vessels," says Dr. Woltering. "If you can stop blood vessel growth, you can stop tumor growth."

Dr. Woltering goes on to say that "all of us (carcinoid specialists) think that we're going to be able to develop a cocktail of medications. Or we'll be able to use 'smart bombs' which are a combination of the right chemotherapy drug and the right anti-angiogenic drug used together."

Part of the problem is money. Research dollars are limited, and most federal dollars go toward more traditional cancer research. Both the Carcinoid Cancer Foundation and The Caring For Carcinoid Foudnation rely heavily on corporate or private donations. Dr. Woltering mentions that Louisiana State University has spent over two million dollars to get a radioactive somatostatin program up and running in New Orleans. They have yet to break even.

Another promising treatment is SIR Spheres. From Sirtex Medical, this treatment involves injecting targeted radioactive microspheres that emit Yttrium 90 into the hepatic artery. SIR-Spheres uses a process known as Selective Internal Radiation Therapy (SIRT). What this means is that the tumors are targeted by the radiation, with most healthy liver tissue remaining unaffected. This treatment was FDA approved in 2002 for colorectal cancer patients with tumor spread to the liver, but physicians are hopeful that the treatment will prove helpful to carcinoid patients as well. A similar treatment is Theraspheres, which uses millions of tiny glass beads containing Yttrium 90 and is injected into the hepatic artery. The results on both of these treatments are promising.

Frequently asked Questions

Is Carcinoid really Cancer?

Yes. Although it is often treated as a benign disease, it is cancer is slow motion. Carcinoid may be cured if the entire primary tumor is removed, but there have been cases of microscopic tumors re-appearing years after an initial surgery.

What are the most common sites for carcinoid cancer to be found?

According to a recent report, the gastrointestinal tract is the most common site for carcinoid tumors to be found. These tumors are frequently found in the small intestine, stomach, and rectum.

But because the cells that carcinoid tumors are created from are found throughout the body, these tumors can be found just about anywhere, including the appendix, the colon, the pancreas and the lungs.

What are some of the symptoms of Carcinoid Cancer?

Symptoms vary from patient to patient, but can include vague abdominal pain, fatigue, flushing, diarrhea, occasionally wheezing, and can even cause damage to heart valves. Many of these symptoms will not occur until the tumor has spread to the liver.

Is treatment the same for all Carcinoid tumors?

A treatment plan for carcinoid tumors should be highly individualized according to the location of the tumor, whether the tumor has metastasized, and whether you currently suffer from Carcinoid Syndrome.

What is Carcinoid Syndrome?

Carcinoid Syndrome is a variety of symptoms from which patients whose primary tumor has metastasized suffer. Those whose primary is in the lung or ovary can also suffer from Carcinoid Syndrome, even without liver metastases. Carcinoid Syndrome is characterized by flushing, diarrhea, wheezing, fatigue, and pain. Carcinoid Syndrome also contributes to additional conditions, such as valvular heart disease, dangerous fluctuations in blood pressure, and a rapid heartbeat.

What is the best way to convince your healthcare professional that you want to be screened for carcinoid?

It's important to remember that some of the many symptoms associated with carcinoid can be present in less serious medical conditions. However, if testing has ruled out the more common ailments, you should certainly suggest to your doctor that you be tested for carcinoid. If for some reason, your doctor refuses, contact one of the 'experts' listed in this book or on the carcinoid.org website. Most of these doctors will work with your local physicians in coordinating your treatment, if in fact your doctor does suspect carcinoid.

How do I find a Carcinoid Specialist?

There are many different ways. Some are listed in this book. You can also contact The Carcinoid Cancer Foundation (www.carcinoid.org) for a more complete list of physicians that specialize in treating carcinoid and other neuroendocrine tumors. Contacting a local carcinoid support group is also a good idea.

GLOSSARY

I have included the definitions of some carcinoid related words that are found throughout the text of this book. I'm grateful to the Carcinoid Cancer Foundation for providing much of this information.

5-HIAA – A breakdown product of serotonin that is excreted in urine. Both serotonin and 5-HIAA are often elevated in carcinoid patients.

ADRENAL GLANDS – Endocrine glands that are found above each kidney, which secretes various hormones like epinephrine and norepinephrine.

BILE – Fluid produced by the liver and stored in the gallbladder that aids in digestion.

CARCINOID – Slow growing tumors, which can be categorized as benign or malignant, or a combination of both (cancer in slow motion.) There are both typical and a-typical carcinoid tumors.

CARCINOID CRISIS – Sudden flushing, and a dangerous change in blood pressure (usually a sudden drop, but can also spike) caused by stress or while under anesthesia.

CARCINOID SYNDROME – A variety of symptoms caused by a tumor producing excessive hormones. Symptoms include flushing, diarrhea, rapid pulse, and sudden change in blood pressure.

CARCINOMA – Malignant tumors that can typically metastasize to various parts of the body. These tumors arise from organs.

CATHETER – A small, hollow tube, which allows fluid passage. It is also used for diagnosing or during specific medical procedures.

CHROMOGRANIN A – A blood tumor marker that is used in screening for various neuroendocrine tumors.

CRYOBLATION – A treatment that is designed to eliminate or reduce tumors by freezing tumors using special instruments.

DEPOT INJECTION – A form of injection that retains the injected substance at the original site so that it is absorbed over an extended period of time.

DIURETIC – A drug used to increase urine flow.

DOPAMINE – A neurotransmitter that is formed in the brain and is necessary for normal central nervous system function.

ENDOCRINE SYSTEM – A series of glands that secrete numerous hormones.

ENDOSCOPE – An instrument that allows visual examination of internal organs such as the stomach and colon.

GASTRIN – Hormones that are secreted in the stomach and regulates gastric acid secretion.

GLUCAGON – A hormone produced by the pancreas that increases blood sugar levels.

HEPATIC ARTERY – The artery that provides 25 percent of the total blood supply to the liver, but 100 percent of the blood supply that nourishes liver tumors.

HEPATIC ARTERY CHEMO-EMBOLIZATION – Using a catheter, chemotherapy drugs are injected directly into the hepatic artery, after which the artery is blocked, thus both eliminating the blood supply to the liver and locking in the chemotherapy drugs.

HISTAMINE – Produced as a reaction to allergens.

HORMONES – A substance produced by certain organs or cells that is carried throughout the bloodstream.

HYPOKALEMIA – Low blood potassium. Normal concentration level is 3.5 to 5.

INSULIN – A hormone that helps regulate metabolism of fat and carbohydrates.

Ki-67 – A biomarker that measures tumor activity.

METASTASES – Spread of cancer cells from original tumor site to various parts of the body.

MRI – Magnetic Resonance Imaging. It produces detailed images of the body by using radio waves and magnets.

NEUROENDOCRINE TUMOR – Tumor derived from cells that release certain hormones in excess.

OCTREO-SCAN® – A scan that requires injection of radioactive octreotide into a vein and subsequently displays all tumor cells in the body that have somatostatin receptors.

OCTREOTIDE ACETATE – Synthetic somatostatin that can inhibit the excess hormones that are produced by various neuroendocrine tumors.

PANCREATIC CARCINOID TUMOR – A carcinoid tumor found on the pancreas; not the same as pancreatic cancer.

PANCREATIC ENZYME – A protein that is secreted in the pancreas and aids in food digestion.

PICC – Peripherally Inserted Central Catheter; a thin, flexible tube that is inserted into a vein in the arm and is used for infusion treatments or to draw blood.

PORT – A small, round disc that attaches to a catheter that is placed just beneath the skin. Usually placed in the chest or abdomen, the attached catheter is inserted into a vein for easy drug or fluid infusion.

PORTAL VEIN – Vein that divides into left and right branches in the liver. 75 percent of blood circulation to the liver is through the portal vein.

POTASSIUM/MAGNESIUM DRIP – A mixture of potassium and magnesium given to a patient via an IV.

RADIOFREQUENCY ABLATION – A form of heat treatment similar to cryoblation, but using heat to kill tumors.

SANDOSTATIN® – Brand name for octreotide acetate.

SANDOSTATIN LAR®– Long-acting version of octreotide acetate given by depot injection.

SEROTONIN – A compound found in the brain, gastric membranes, and blood serum. Levels are often elevated in carcinoid patients.

SIR SPHERES – Radioactive microspheres that emit Yttrium 90 and are injected directly into the hepatic artery.

SOMATOSTATIN ANALOGS – Standard treatment for carcinoid patients. They include octreotide, lanreotide, and vapreotide.

SUBCUTANEOUS – Just beneath the skin.

THERASPHERES – A procedure that uses tiny glass beads to inject radiation directly into the tumors using Yttrium 90.

TINCTURE OF OPIUM – Opiate used to slow the chronic diarrhea often seen in carcinoid patients.

TPN – Total Parental Nutrition; often given to patients who can no longer digest food. TPN does not utilize the digestive system.

TUMOR DEBULKING – The surgical procedure that removes as much of the existing tumors as possible.

VIP – Vasoactive Intestinal Polypeptide.

EPILOGUE

Today, even with medical advances, carcinoid cancer continues to claim the life of too many people. Yet the future holds promise for those who continue to suffer with this misunderstood disease.

My life has changed forever since the death of my sister. There have been days that I have been unable to look at the words I've written in this book, because they remind me of the pain and struggles that Marge went through. There are days that I read about new, cutting-edge treatments and I get excited, but it's always tempered by a lasting sense of regret that Marge cannot benefit from any of those treatments.

Marge and I both thought that she would live to see a cure for carcinoid cancer. It is now my hope that those currently suffering from this disease, along with those yet to be diagnosed will be able to benefit from these exciting developments and we will one day be able to put 'carcinoid' on the list of 'curable' diseases.

I often play the 'what if' game. It's a game that we're all familiar with. I think things like "*What if Marge had seen one of the carcinoid specialists? What if she had begun treatment soon after her tumor was discovered? What if she had seen a doctor who was more aggressive?*"

No one can answer any of those questions. And even if they could, the outcome would remain the same.

In November 2004, just two months after Marge's death, I had the privilege to speak with Dr. Eugene Woltering and Dr. Lowell Anthony, two of the top carcinoid specialists in the world. Both were gracious and willing to spend some of their valuable time answering my questions. Of course, the subject often returned to Marge. Trying to make some sense out of her death, I confided to Dr. Woltering that I wished that Marge had been able to consult with him.

His response surprised me. "Maybe the ten years she lived after surgery was a gift. Maybe she would have been one of those patients who develop complications after surgery. Maybe she lived ten years more because she didn't have more aggressive treatment."

When I left Dr. Woltering's office, I continued to replay his words in my head. We all know that when a loved one is terminally ill, no amount of time left together is ever enough. If we have five months, we want a year. If we have ten years, we want ten more. But I know, when that old resentment rises in me, and I wish for all of those things that I cannot possibly have, I now think of Dr. Woltering's words. And I'm thankful for those ten years. I'm thankful that Marge was able to have a good life, albeit a short one. I'm thankful that she was able to meet and love my son Jared. I'm thankful that she lived her life the way she wanted to, and I believe even died the same way.

I still wish it could have been more.

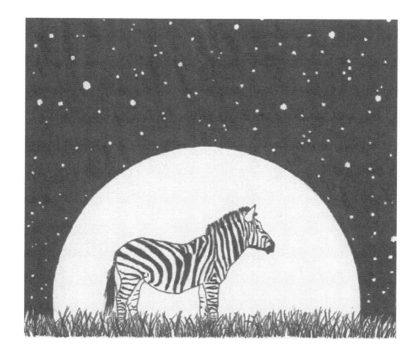

MY STORY

By Margaret A. Durlak

It all began one fall night in 1985. I had been out with a friend for dinner. That night when I went to bed, a pain unlike any I had ever experienced shot through my stomach. I got up, took an antacid and tried to go back to sleep, but that didn't work. I was up most of the night in pain. By morning the pain had gone. I figured it was just something I ate. I was okay after that for some time, maybe three months or so. Then one night the pain came back. I'm not one to go to a doctor unless it's absolutely necessary. Being the procrastinator that I am, it was quite some time before I would finally seek the opinion of a doctor.

The doctor I saw was a stomach specialist, so I assumed my pain would be taken care of. I was sent for an upper GI, but the results came back normal. I was told to avoid spicy foods, not to eat too late at night and of course lose some weight. Well, I tried all of those things, even losing weight, but the pain returned.

Things went on like this for sometime. I was beginning to think I was crazy or just imagining this pain. So I sought out the advice of a different doctor. I thought that the problem could be my Gallbladder. I explained all of my symptoms to him and mentioned this. He didn't think so, and without any testing, ended up giving me the same advice as the first doctor, along with a prescription for Prilosec. The medication didn't help and the pain was still there. I made another appointment, this time requesting an Ultrasound of the Gallbladder. Nothing! This time I was told to raise the head of my bed, sleep on my right side and of course lose more weight. I've been overweight for most of my life, so I didn't think being FAT could cause this much pain or that this was the root of my problem. But that seemed to be every doctor's answer. I resigned myself to the fact that this pain was just something I was going to have to live with.

Soon the pain was happening more often and with more intensity. I was vomiting and had frequent bowel movements. I was unable to eat or drink anything for at least a 24-hour period. One thing was certain; I was losing weight.

In 1992 I started keeping a log of when I would get these attacks and how long they lasted. I began to see a pattern. The pain seemed to occur around my menstrual cycle. I went to see my gynecologist with this new information. She did an exam but didn't think this had anything to do with my cycle and referred me to an Internist

Once again I was telling my story to a new doctor. However this doctor didn't suggest I lose weight or sleep on my right side. She scheduled me for an MRI. The MRI revealed a mass in my pancreas.

I was relieved to find out that there was a reason for all this pain and illness. But at the same time I was scared as hell. I went for a CT scan and then a biopsy was done. The biopsy showed both normal and abnormal cells. My Internist suggested I see a surgeon.

The surgeon looked at the test results, and then explained the procedure he would perform if I chose to have surgery. He would make a small incision, take a piece of the mass and have it analyzed during surgery. If the cells were found to be "normal" he would proceed with the removal of the mass.

Before having surgery, I wanted a second opinion. So I gathered all of my records and went to see another surgeon at a large hospital in Chicago. After reviewing my records and seeing my CT scan, the surgeon was sure he could remove the mass. He drew a diagram explaining what he was going to do and how he would resection my stomach. He scheduled the surgery and told me "If you've had this pain since 1985 and this were a malignant tumor, we would not be here talking about it." Made sense to me.

So there I was at the hospital at 6:00 AM with my father and boyfriend, Jesse, waiting to go into surgery. As I said my good-byes, I knew in my gut that this tumor would still be with me after surgery.

I was right. I woke up in recovery at 1:30pm and heard someone on the phone, trying to get a bed for me. I fell back asleep and woke again at 3:00pm. I listened as the nurse gave a change of shift report, explaining to her replacement about the surgery that had been done and that "the tumor was not removed." With that, out I went!

When I woke again around 5:30pm; they were finally taking me to a room. As they wheeled me down the hall I saw my Dad and Jesse. Neither one of them looked too well at that point. So when I finally got in the bed I asked Jesse, "Am I dying?" He said no, and with that I told him to "get the f…ng look off his face and take my dad and go home!"

The next day the surgeon came in and told me he was sorry that he could not remove the tumor. He said a few other things that I could not recall, but from the gist of the conversation it seemed that I should start shopping for a casket. The surgeon made an appointment for me to see an oncologist that specialized in pancreatic tumors. That alone terrified me. I spent that next week thinking nothing but the worst. When I finally met the oncologist, Dr. S, I felt much better. He explained to me that if the tumor showed growth that I would need to undergo chemotherapy.

My next CT scan was approximately 2 months after the first one. There was no change in the size of the tumor, which was about the size of an orange. I had to see the surgeon one more time to be released back to work. That was the last time I saw him.

The rest of my treatment would be handled by Dr. S. and his office. My care was then put in the hands of Dr. A, who was doing his fellowship under Dr. S's direction. I saw him the year following my surgery with visits and CT scans every three months. There was no change in the tumor.

About a year after surgery, I began having very unusual diarrhea, not often, but not normal. Procrastinating again, I didn't mention it. At the end of the year Dr. A's fellowship was over and he was moving on to his own practice in another part of the state. This concerned me, as I had grown comfortable with the treatment I was receiving. Little did I know that on my next visit I would meet the doctor that would be able to diagnose and treat my disease.

My next visit would be with Dr. G. When it was time for my CT scan and visit I was a little nervous, not knowing anything about this new doctor. When I finally met him, most of my worries disappeared. He had my chart but asked that I tell him about my problem. So here I was explaining my story to yet another person. But I liked him and I had a feeling this new doctor would be "OK." He called me a few days later to let me know my CT was unchanged.

Within a few weeks of my visit, my unusual diarrhea was increasing. Now it was accompanied by nausea and it was becoming difficult for me to stay awake. I was losing strength and my muscles were beginning to hurt, which made it difficult to walk or climb stairs. Dr. G prescribed some medication for the nausea but it didn't seem to help. This went on for nearly a month. I was losing weight and beginning to get a bit nervous. In September alone, I lost 45 pounds.

Dr. G had an idea of what may be causing the diarrhea. To be sure, I had to do a 24-hour urine test. Prior to the 24-hour urine, he mentioned a medication that would be able to control the diarrhea. I told him I would take any thing. Then he told me the only way to take the medication was by subcutaneous injection. This hit me hard. I never imagined that I would be taking daily injections for anything!

In the mean time, I had no appetite and nothing could quench my thirst. I was talking to my sister who lived in Las Vegas at the time, letting her know about this problem I was having. Her husband, whom I had yet to meet (they were married in February, this was September) suggested that

I try Gatorade, which worked. (I later found out this probably saved my life.) Two days later I returned to find out what my urine test revealed. I was diagnosed with a "VIPoma" tumor. VIP is a hormone produced by the body.

The following week, I could barely stay awake or walk. It happened to be a busy day at the clinic and I had a very long wait to see Dr. G. By the time he came into the examining room I was laying on the desk, almost asleep. He confirmed his findings and was taking me down to the chemotherapy lab to have a nurse show me how to use the needle. When I got up to follow him I could barely walk. He asked what was wrong; I told him my legs hurt. While in the lab he had blood drawn. I sat with the nurse as she showed me how to use the needle. It was a long ride home.

The next day was my dad's 75th birthday and I had planned a party for him. There were several errands to run, so this was a very difficult day for me. I had no energy but knew things had to be done. By the time I got home from my errands, I collapsed on the couch. I was not able to move. My dad became very concerned, calling my name often to see if I was ok. I was able to respond, but just couldn't bring myself to move. I laid on the couch from 11 AM to approximately 6 PM when my boyfriend, Jesse came home. I heard the phone ring, and then Jesse came to tell me the call was for me. He helped me from the couch to the phone. On the line was a doctor calling on behalf of my doctor. She said that my blood test came back, my potassium was low and Dr. G wanted me to come to the hospital ER. I asked her when.

"Right now," she responded. I asked how low my potassium was. She told me 1.75. I had no idea that was dangerously low. So I sat with my dad and our guests while they ate the dinner I should have prepared, but my dad ended up preparing.

Some party!

I packed a few things in the event they would keep me, and then we left for the hospital. The doctor told me that the ER would be expecting me. When I got there, I filled out a few papers and waited a short time then was taken into the ER. Once in there I met with a doctor who asked me to explain what my problem was. After telling him, he checked my reflexes.   I don't think I had any in my right knee. He then asked me to pull his fingers as hard as I could. As I was pulling, he told me to "pull as hard as you can."

I told him I was pulling as hard as I can. The next thing I knew he pulled back the curtain and started shouting orders. (I felt like I was in a scene from ER). I was given orange juice with some type of potassium, an IV was inserted and an EKG was done. They told me I would be spending the night. So, I had my boyfriend come into the room to let him know I was staying and that he should go home.

When I was being brought to my room, I noticed the sign that said 'WELCOME TO THE CARDIAC UNIT.' I asked the nurse why I was on a cardiac unit and he told me that with my potassium being so low my heart could have stopped. I had no clue I was so sick.

I was in the hospital for four days. They pumped approximately fifteen bags of potassium chloride into me. When they removed the IV on the day of my discharge, my entire body seemed to swell up, especially my legs. It would take a week before my body would go back to normal. At that time I was taking one injection of 50mcg octreotide. Once I was home, I had to administer the drug myself without any supervision. The first day was very difficult. The pharmacy gave me the wrong size syringes, and I had to give myself two injections. I contacted the pharmacy and they were able to exchange the syringes for the correct size. This procedure took some time to get use to. But it made me feel so much better that it was worth it. About three months later I began feeling sluggish and tired again, so Dr. G increased my dosage to 100 mcg per injection. This helped immediately. I would continue to use this dose from September of 1995 to April of 1999.   Then I began getting the same sluggish feeling and experiencing some diarrhea again. It turned out that my potassium had once again dropped. I now began taking two injections per day of 100 mcg of octreotide, and a potassium supplement twice a day.

This helped to increase my potassium level and the octreotide helped to decrease my diarrhea. I was able to function again. Somewhere in the year 2000, the same old feeling came back again. So I decided to do some experimenting of my own. I started giving myself an extra injection. This meant I was now taking 100 mcg three times a day. This seemed to help greatly. I then contacted Dr G's office and asked him to rewrite my prescription. After a visit to the office, he was able to increase my dosage. It remained this way throughout 2000, 2001 and most of 2002. All this time I have regularly scheduled CT scans to monitor my tumor.

I found out in the early part of 2002 that my doctor would no longer accept my health insurance which meant I would have to find a new doctor to continue my care. I located a doctor in Chicago at a large teaching hospital .I was scheduled to see Dr. *** for the first time in July.

In April of 2002, I had my usual and last CT scan at the other hospital. About three weeks later, I received a call from Dr. G informing me that there were new lesions on my liver and he thought I would now benefit from chemotherapy. Let me say this totally blew me away. I was also scheduled to see my new Oncologist in July. I saw Dr. G for the last time in June and decided to wait until my appointment with Dr. *** before making any decisions. Let me tell you, this put me into something of a panic. I would be leaving the one doctor that knew what was wrong with me. If I haven't mentioned it as yet, this is a very rare type of cancer.

Once I met with Dr. *** I liked him immediately. It was very reassuring to talk to a doctor that knew more about my illness then I did. He decided to put me thru a complete battery of tests including another CT scan. But during this initial period my diarrhea became very severe and I ended up having two separate potassium infusions. I began having my potassium level checked every three to five days, and also began taking additional supplements of potassium (K-DUR) seven times daily. In addition, I was taking Lomotil, to help slow the diarrhea four times daily and a pancreatic enzyme to help in digestion. My octreotide was increased to 300mcg three times a day, and I was given a diuretic to help eliminate the extra fluid in my legs being caused by the large quantities of K-Dur I was taking. Needless to say it was a long summer.

It's now late 2002 and I am scheduled to see Dr. *** soon. We will schedule my next CT Scan and go from there. One thing he did tell me was that he did not think I had a VIPoma. He was convinced it was a pancreatic carcinoid.

Of late I am feeling good. I have occasional bouts of diarrhea and my potassium is up and down. But I am able to handle it.

I am thankful for many things. I now have a doctor that is able to understand what I go through on a daily basis. I have a job I enjoy. I have friends that are of great support to me. And I have my family, who without their help I may have gone long ago.

AUTHOR'S NOTES

March 13, 2007

At 2:00 AM Pacific time, The Stardust Hotel and Casino in Las Vegas, Nevada was imploded. It's impossible for me to imagine Las Vegas without The Stardust: it held center court for so many of the events that took place in our lives, some of which I've touched on in *Carcinoid Cancer, Zebras and Stardust.*

Yet in retrospect, the demise of The Stardust seems almost fitting. It would never be the same without Marge.

Psychic Sylvia Browne says that in Heaven you are surrounded by the places that you love the most, so I'm pretty sure I know where Marge is spending her time these days. The thought reassures me that maybe, one day, we'll be able to be together again at the place that has meant so much to both of us.

I know that as The Stardust disappeared from the Las Vegas Strip for eternity, and the dust rose to the heavens, a tall, pretty blonde stood ready to welcome the arrival of a beloved friend with open arms.

Viva Las Vegas, Marge.

— Mary Girsch-Bock – March 2007

IMPORTANT UPDATES

CLINICAL TRIALS

There have been several significant clinical trials undertaken in the last few years that continue to bring hope to neuroendocrine tumor sufferers. A clinical trial using Lithium in the treatment of low-grade neuroendocrine tumors was completed at the University of Wisconsin, with results of the trial pending. Phase II of a study to determine the safety of Atiprimod, an anti-proliferative, anti-angiogenic drug in Advanced Carcinoid Cancer Patients was recently undertaken. The University of California, San Francisco is currently conducting a clinical trial with Bevacizumab, which is a monoclonal antibody that is designed to stop tumor growth by preventing the formation of new blood vessels that typically feed the tumor. Some researchers believe that using Bevacizumab with combination chemotherapeutic agents such as 5-fluorouracil, leucovorin, and oxaliplatin may inhibit tumor growth more effectively than using either therapy separately. A study completed in 2007 by The Clinical Science Center in Madison, Wisconsin studied the effectiveness of valproic acid (VPA), a drug that is commonly used in epilepsy. Treatment was conducted on both gastrointestinal and pulmonary carcinoid cells, and resulted in a dose-dependent inhibition of cancer cell growth.

Clinical studies remain focused on molecularly targeted and anti-angiogenic therapies, with more hospitals and clinics participating than ever before.

NEW TREATMENT

The FDA approved the use of Lutetieum-177 radionuclide, labeled with Octreotate. Lutetium -177 Octreotate is a somatostatin receptor seeking agent that can detect neuroendocrine tumor cells throughout the body, attach to them and deliver therapeutic doses of radioactivity directly to the tumor. This targeted radionuclide therapy has shown significant therapeutic effect on previously progressive tumors, providing targeted treatment to the tumors. Excel Diagnostics and Nuclear Oncology Center in Houston, Texas is the first facility in the United States to offer this therapy. The treatment has been used in Europe for over 10 years, and is currently available in Australia and India as well.

The trials and treatment described above are just the beginning of more targeted therapies designed for those with neuroendocrine tumors that typically have a low response rate when subjected to traditional chemotherapy. For all of those suffering from a neuroendocrine tumor, or know someone who is, more aggressive therapies and cutting-edge clinical trials bring a new dose of hope that one day this cancer can be controlled, and eventually eradicated. In the meantime, individual, aggressive treatment plans, and targeted therapies will work to improve quality of life and extend survival rates significantly.

REFERENCES

INTRODUCTION

Woltering, Eugene "Introduction to the Basic Science of Carcinoid"
Carcinoid Wellness Center – New Orleans, LA (2002)
www.carcinoid.org/nociwolt.htm

CHAPTER TWO

Warner, Richard R.P., "A Review of Carcinoid Cancer"
Carcinoid Cancer Foundation (2005)
www.carcinoid.org/pcf/docs/review.html

Zuetenhorst, Johanna, M., and Taal, Babs G., "Metastatic Carcinoid Tumors: A Clinical Review" The Oncologist (2005) 10:123-131

Ardill, JES, and Erikkson, B., "The Importance of the Measurement of Circulating Markers in Patients with Neuroendocrine Tumours of the Pancreas and Gut." Endocrine – Related Cancer (2003) 10: 459-462

Holdcroft, A., "Hormones and the Gut" British Journal of Anaesthesia (2000) 85:58-68

Comaru-Schally, Anna Maria, and Schally, Andrew V., "A Clinical Overview of Carcinoid Tumors: Perspectives for Improvement in Treatment Using Peptide Analogs (Review)" International Journal of Oncology (2005) 26:301-309

Warner, Richard R.P., "A Review of Carcinoid Cancer" Carcinoid Cancer Foundation (2005) www.carcinoid.org/pcf/docs/review.html

CHAPTER THREE

Anthony, Lowell – "Transcript from Interview – New Orleans, LA" (2004)

Barakat, M.T., Meeran, K., and Bloom, S.R., "Neuroendocrine Tumors" Endocrine – Related Cancer (2004) 11:1-18

Vinik, Aaron, I "Clinical Aspects of Neuroendocrine Tumors" Carcinoid/NET Conference – Philadelphia, PA 2005

Warner, Richard, R. P., "Carcinoid Tumors and Carcinoid Syndrome" Carcinoid Cancer Foundation (2003) www.carcinoid.org./warner/lectureoct2503.htm

Warner, Richard R.P., "A Review of Carcinoid Cancer" Carcinoid Cancer Foundation (2005) www.carcinoid.org/pcf/docs/review.html

CHAPTER FOUR

Warner, Richard R.P., "A Review of Carcinoid Cancer" Carcinoid Cancer Foundation (2005) www.carcinoid.org/pcf/docs/review.html

CHAPTER EIGHT

Comaru-Schally, Anna Maria, and Schally, Andrew V., "A Clinical Overview of Carcinoid Tumors: Perspectives for Improvement in Treatment Using Peptide Analogs" (Review) International Journal of Oncology (2005) 26:301-309

CHAPTER ELEVEN

Woltering M.D., Eugene – "Transcript from Interview – New Orleans, LA" (2004)

CHAPTER TWELVE

Anthony M.D., Lowell – "Transcript from Interview – New Orleans, LA "(2004)

Woltering M.D., Eugene – "Transcript from Interview – New Orleans, LA" (2004)

Warner, Richard R.P., "A Review of Carcinoid Cancer" Carcinoid Cancer Foundation (2005) www.carcinoid.org/pcf/docs/review.html

CHAPTER THIRTEEN

Pommier, Rodney "The Role of Surgery and Chemoembolization in the Management of Carcinoid" California Carcinoid Fighters Conference (2003)

The National Center for Biotechnology Information "What Is a Cell?" (NCBI) 2004 http://www.ncbi.nih.gov/about/primer/genetics_cell.html

Warner, Richard R.P., "A Review of Carcinoid Cancer" Carcinoid Cancer Foundation (2005) www.carcinoid.org/pcf/docs/review.html

Woltering M.D., Eugene – "Transcript from Interview – New Orleans, LA" (2004)

RadiologyInfo.org "Chemboembolization" (2005)
www.radiologyinfo.org

Society of Interventional Radiology "Cancer Treatment"
www.sirweb.org/patpub/livercancertreatment/shtml
(2006)

RadiologyInfo.org "Radiofrequency Ablation of Liver Tumors" (2005)
www.radiologyinfo.org

FREQUENTLY ASKED QUESTIONS

Anthony M.D., Lowell – "Transcript from Interview – New Orleans, LA "(2004)

Öberg, Kjell, "Diagnosis and Treatment of Carcinoid Tumors" Expert Rev. Anticancer Therapy 3 (6) (2003)

Warner, Richard R.P., "A Review of Carcinoid Cancer" Carcinoid Cancer Foundation (2005)
www.carcinoid.org/pcf/docs/review.html

Woltering M.D., Eugene – Transcript from Interview – New Orleans

NEW DEVELOPMENTS

Greenblatt DY, Vaccaro AM, Jaskilua-Sztul R, Ning L, Haymart M, Kunnimalaiyaan M, Chen H "Valproic Acid Activates Notch-1 Signaling and Regulates the Neuroendocrine Phenotype in Carcinoid Cancer Cells" Oncologist. 2007 Aug;12 (8):942-51

ABOUT THE BOOK

Carcinoid Cancer, Zebras and Stardust is the story of one person's relentless battle against carcinoid, and of the author's struggle to come to terms with the death of her beloved sister.

Inside, you'll also find the words of some of the world's top carcinoid specialists, invaluable reference data, and a comprehensive list of the top carcinoid specialists.

ABOUT THE AUTHOR

Mary Girsch-Bock was born and raised in the Chicagoland area, and still considers Chicago "home."

After a career in the healthcare and property management industries, Mary began a successful freelance writing career, specializing in business and technology issues, and is currently a contributing writer for *The CPA Technology Advisor*.

Mary began researching carcinoid tumors shortly after her sister Marge's diagnosis in 1995, and continues to do so today.

Shortly before her death, Marge conveyed her desire to have her story told. From that desire came "Of Zebras and Stardust."

Mary currently lives in the Southwest with her husband Shannon, son Jared, three birds, and a neurotic dog.

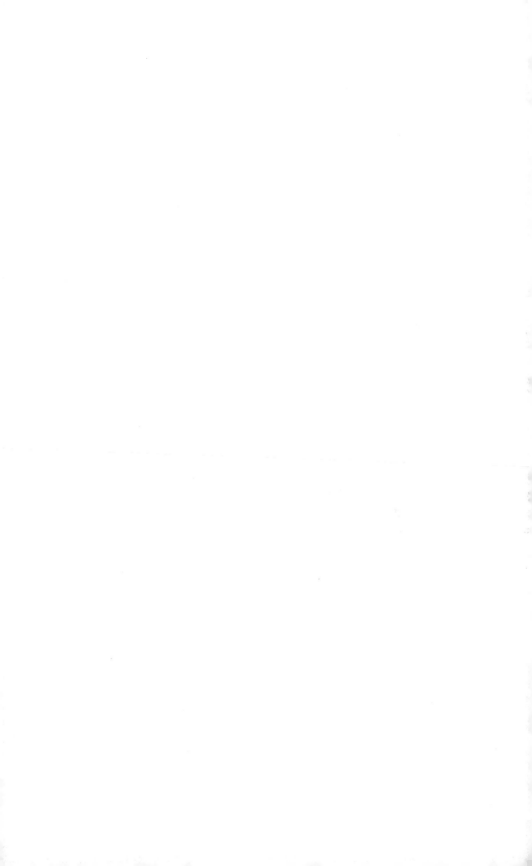